Basic Concepts in Statistics and Epidemiology

Théodore H MacDonald

Professor (Emeritus), Associate of the Research Institute of Human Rights and Social Justice at London Metropolitan University

Foreword by
Allyson Pollock

Radcliffe Publishing
Oxford • San Francisco

Radcliffe Publishing Ltd
18 Marcham Road
Abingdon
Oxon OX14 1AA
United Kingdom

www.radcliffe-oxford.com
Electronic catalogue and worldwide online ordering facility.

British Library Cataloguing in Publication Data

A catalogue record for this book is available from the British Library.

ISBN-10: 1 84619 124 6
ISBN-13: 978 1 84619 124 4

Typeset by Anne Joshua & Associates, Oxford, UK
Printed and bound by Biddles Ltd, King's Lynn, Norfolk, UK

Contents

Foreword   **vii**

Preface   **viii**

Acknowledgements   **x**

1   **Describing a mass of data**   **1**
Population samples and scores   1
Distributions   1
Two basic types of measure   5
Measures of central tendency   6
Measures of dispersion   7
Grouped data   11
Study exercises   18
Study exercises 1   18

2   **A necessary glimpse of probability**   **20**
The problem of statistical inference   20
Some basic laws of probability   21
Probability in health calculations   23
Binomials raised to various powers   26
Permutations   29
Factorial notation   31
Calculating with permutations   32
Combinations   34
Repeated trials   36
Study exercises 2   40

3   **Using the normal curve**   **42**
Parametric statistical analysis   42
Normal distribution   42
When the infinite is finite   44
Relating σ to probabilities   46

4   **An approximation to the normal curve**   **50**
The binomial distribution   50
Throwing dice   50

Approximating the normal curve   52
Using the binomial distribution algebraically   54
Testing statistical hypotheses   58
The relationship between binomial and normal distributions   60

5   **Testing samples**   **62**
Random samples   63
Study exercises 3   64
Testing a sample   65
Analysing a test of sample mean   67
The null hypothesis   67
Looking at sample means more intuitively   70
Testing a difference of means of large samples   73
Confidence limits   75
Study exercises 4   76

6   **Testing small samples**   **77**
Problems with small samples   77
Two samples   77
The t-test   78
Actually calculating 't'   80
Another application of the t-distribution   81
Establishing an interval for the population mean   83
Comparing a sample mean with the population mean   84
Why demand equal standard deviations?   85

7   **A taste of epidemiology**   **86**
What is epidemiology?   86
Various proportions and rates   86
Sensitivity, specificity and predictive value   88
More informed sectioning of probability spaces   89
Joint probability   89
Conditional probability   91
Dependent and independent events   92
Application to disease states   93
Apparent anomalies   95
Study exercises 5   96

8   **From Binomial to Poisson**   **98**
Rates of occurrence   98
Exponential growth and decay   99
Natural growth and 'e'   100
The general formula for Compound Interest   102
Changing to natural growth   104

Evaluating 'e'   105
Link between rate and risk   107
Poisson distribution   109
Death by horse kick   111
The Poisson and binomial distribution compared   111

9 Non-parametric statistics   **112**
What is 'non-parametric'?   112
Wilcoxon two-independent sample test   112
The sign test for the paired case   116
The Wilcoxon test for the paired case   118
The chi-square test   121
Study exercises 6   128

10 For the algebraically innocent   **130**
Measuring correlations   130
Straight line equations   130
Locating points   131
Graphing algebraic expressions   132
Straight lines and their gradients   135
Calculating a straight line's slope   135
Going from graph to algebra   138
Study exercises 7   139

11 The Gini coefficient   **141**
The non-clinical context of health   141
The Lorenz curve explained   141
The Gini coefficient   142
Gini coefficients worldwide   143
Strengths of G as a measure of income inequality   146
Critical comments on the use of G-score   147

12 Correlation: a measure of relatedness   **149**
Are they cor-related or co-related?   149
Computing a value for correlation   150
The Pearson product-moment correlation coefficient   154
How about remembering formulae?   155
Calculating r from grouped data   156
Remarks about r 158
The sampling distribution of r-scores   159

13 The problem of prediction   **161**
Linear correlation   161
Back to the algebra   163

Where to from here?   165
Study exercises 8   166

14 Introducing ANOVA   **167**
What can ANOVA do for you?   167
Assumptions underlying ANOVA   169
Developing procedures for ANOVA   171
What do the two variances mean?   173
Setting up the variance table   175
Discussion of steps in ANOVA   175
An ANOVA problem   178
But why use ANOVA?   180

15 A brief introduction to designing a research project   **182**
Formulating your research problem   182
Writing up the proposal   184
Revising, doing, revising   185

Answers to study exercises   **186**

Appendix A Areas under the normal probability curve (Z-table) 190

Appendix B Distribution of t 192

Appendix C Wilcoxon distribution (with no pairing)   193

Appendix D Wilcoxon distribution (with pairing) where $W_1 \leq n$ 195

Appendix E Wilcoxon distribution (with pairing) where $W_1 > n$ 196

Appendix F Random numbers   198

Appendix G Transformation of r to z 200

Appendix H Poisson values   202

Appendix I χ^2 Values   204

Appendix J F-values   206

Index   207

Foreword

This little book will be a great primer for all students and research workers engaged in learning how to use statistical ideas in public health. It sets out the core concepts and explains them clearly, using worked examples as illustration. If followed carefully, the engaged reader should be able to use the standard statistical software packages intelligently and sensitively. As Professor MacDonald points out, statistics are often abused and misinterpreted because the users do not fully understand the implications of probabilistic inference. The plethora of convenient statistics software packages beg better usage. Wrongly applied, they can become lethal instruments in the hands of policy makers or, indeed, even of medical witnesses in courts of law.

Association, causation, probability, risk and prediction are important concepts in the sciences of healthcare and medical research. Clinicians and researchers need to be able to understand basic epidemiology and how the incidence and prevalence of disease relate to the general population. But they also need to communicate to their patients how such things as the probability of passing on an inherited disorder, the risks of contracting an infectious disease and the probability of death, morbidity or cure following treatment are calculated. To be able to critically appraise medical research, to assess the statistics and science behind clinical trials, and to evaluate the efficacy of health services are essential skills. This little primer on the rationale underlying the basics constitutes an excellent starting point. It is to be hoped that it will stimulate the public health student, in whatever context, and new researchers to approach the enterprise with enhanced confidence in interpreting and coherently explaining their findings.

Professor Allyson Pollock
Centre of International Public Health Policy
University of Edinburgh
November 2006

Preface

Medical, and other healthcare teaching and research relies heavily on the use of statistics, inferences based on probability theory and on epidemiology. Research workers, and students, have traditionally experienced difficulty in understanding the bases on which their statistical and other calculations are founded. In an attempt to meet their needs in this respect, most institutions running undergraduate and graduate programmes in the health disciplines routinely include a compulsory module on statistics and/or research methods.

Anyone who has taught such modules soon realises that the amount of specific detail required is far too great to cover in sufficient intellectual depth in the time allocated, for the students to develop a firm grasp of what is really happening. The many fine computer statistics packages – software into which students and researchers can feed their data for statistical analysis – are being increasingly employed in an attempt to meet the challenge. But, over many years of experience in teaching research methods, in supervising postgraduate research and in serving on the editorial boards of various health journals, I have come to realise that very often people engaged in medical research (either as students or as professionals) do not have cognitive insight into the methods used and are thus often lacking in confidence in correctly interpreting the results they obtain.

The standard compulsory module in statistics and research methods, because it is taken in isolation – sometimes even in a different year from that in which students require it to analyse their own data – sometimes renders cognitive insight more difficult. At the same time, the computer packages seem to satisfy the need for data analysis without actually generating sufficient real insight to understand the findings.

Over the last 15 years, I have felt that the solution resides in a series of lessons in which the basic ideas of statistical and probabalistic inference, with respect to health research, are systematically explained. Accordingly the material in this book has been elaborated and trialled in undergraduate and postgraduate classes in the UK, the US and Australia, both by myself and other tutors, since 1990. Over that time changes have been made. At first it was thought that students would not welcome problems set at the end of chapters as they would be anxious to work on their own data. To an extent this turned out to be true, but with some topics – particularly probability – it was found that problem sets (with answers for the probability questions) encouraged participation and discussion, as well as greatly enhancing confidence. Answers are not provided for *every* Study exercise problem as I have found that class discussion of the attempts made is of great value in developing analytic power. Whether any given tutor chooses to use any problem sets provided is best left up to them. Again, not every class will want to do every chapter. Chapters 1–4 are so fundamental that students need a good grasp of that material if they subsequently wish to make intelligent and effective use of computer packages. Likewise, Chapters 5 and 6 explain basic cognitive issues. Many students and tutors very much welcomed Chapter 10 (a review of the basic algebra underlying linear graphs), especially as it rendered the concept of correlations so easy to understand (Chapter 12).

The other chapters provide further insight but might not be essential to the student being able to use the computer statistical packages confidently. Chapters 7 (A taste of epidemiology) and 15 (A brief introduction to designing a research project) tend to be useful to students in public health and/or those who are drawing up a research project. Chapters devoted to topics such as the Poisson distribution, non-parametric statistics (including chi-square), regression lines (prediction) and ANOVA might simply be referred to at a further stage of a student's development as a researcher. They are included for completion. The material included here has been welcomed by tutors in statistics and research methods in various institutions.

Finally, it should be stated that in this account I have confined my attention to quantitative analysis. Qualitative analysis has an increasingly important role to play in interview-based research in public health, but the student with a sound grasp of inferential statistics based on quantitative data can readily learn the many useful approaches to handling the wide variety of data thrown up by qualitative data with their own tutor and as specifically required by the research in question.

Théodore H MacDonald
November 2006

Acknowledgements

Many more people have contributed to this work than I can name. In particular, I refer to the 400+ postgraduate coursework students in universities, colleges, medical schools, etc., in Africa, Australia, Fiji, the USA and the UK on whom the material has been trialled and refined for the past 20 years or so. Without their forbearance, the task would have never been undertaken. A huge debt of gratitude, however, must go to Dr Adam Spargo, a bioinformatician at the Wellcome Trust Sanger Institute. It was he who undertook the thoroughly unenviable task of word processing the manuscript, with all of its unforgiving mathematical symbols, charts, tables and figures. I thank him deeply for his good humour and patience. Then there is, as always, my wonderful wife, Chris, whose moral support throughout the whole authorship process has been my mainstay.

As usual, my copy editors at Radcliffe publishing have been enormously helpful.

The author alone is responsible for any shortcomings in the content.

Chapter 1

Describing a mass of data

Population samples and scores

Health research can generate a great mass of data, only a few scores or something inbetween. In the next three sections we shall deal with the situation in which we have largish quantities of data to deal with – anywhere from, say, 50 to millions.

You probably appreciate that 'data' is a plural, its singular being 'datum'. Typically, each datum (or *score*, as it is usually called in statistics) is a number. The whole set of possible scores that an enquiry can give is called the *population*. Of course, you must realise that only very rarely do we record the whole population. For instance, you might be considering *Clostridium* (a bacterium) counts in tinned carrots of a particular brand. You cannot test every tin of carrots. Instead, you might pick, say 5000 tins, as a *sample* and test each of them. There are certain restrictions on what you can safely conclude about a population from samples taken from it, but in dealing with large masses of data we must know what these restrictions are, for that is basically what we do in statistically analysing populations. We take a sample and do measurements on that.

Distributions

The word 'distribution' describes the general 'shape' of the mass of data. This becomes especially noticeable if we graph the data in some way. Generally, the horizontal axis (usually called the x-axis or abscissa) displays the possible scores, while the scale on the vertical axis (usually called the y-axis or ordinate) indicates how many times each score occurs – the *frequency* of each score.

The following diagrams (Figures 1.1–1.9) indicate some common types of distribution. D^ which allows intermediate measures is *continuous* and it is legitimate graph their distributions with curves.

.ample – blood haemoglobin level. Your points on the x-axis might go: 4, 4.5, 5, 5.5, 6, 6.5, . . . , 15, 15.5, 16; but it is possible to get a reading such as

9.73, which would suggest that its frequency can be indicated by a section of the curve running between x-values 9.5 and 10.0.

On the other hand, some data are such that a curve is meaningless. Take a distribution of mothers according to numbers of live babies to which they have given birth. For instance, some mothers might have produced 4 live babies and some 5. No mothers have produced 4.8 live babies; so it would be senseless to draw an arc of a curve between the frequency points for 4 and 5! Such data is referred to as *discrete* or not continuous (or discontinuous).

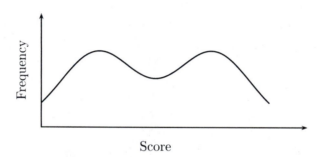

Figure 1.1 This is a bimodal distribution. There is a relatively high frequency of fairly low scores and of fairly high scores, and a relatively low frequency of middle-range scores.

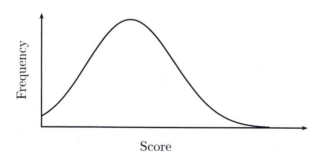

Figure 1.2 Negatively skewed – 'squashed' to the left.

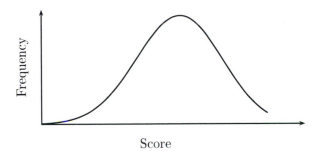

Figure 1.3 Positively skewed – 'squashed' to the right.

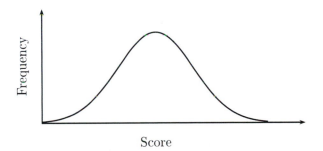

Figure 1.4 Normal distribution – much more about that later! Not all 'bell-shaped' curves are 'normal'.

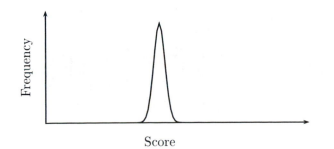

Figure 1.5 Leptokurtotic – a high-pointed, narrow-based distribution. These tend to have small standard deviations (discussed later). Kurtosis refers to 'peakedness'.

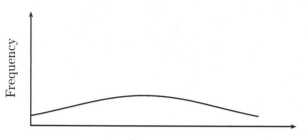

Figure 1.6 Platykurtotic – a flat wide-based distribution. Their standard deviations are bigger. A platypus has a flat mouth, so it is easy to remember that platy means flat.

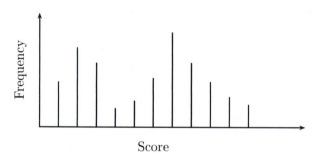

Figure 1.7 A bar graph – particularly suitable for discrete data (data which is not continuous). This is explained below.

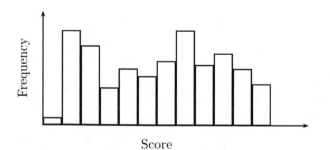

Figure 1.8 Histogram – also good for indicating the shape of a distribution of discrete data. The actual scores occur at the midpoint of the base of each rectangle. Their frequencies are indicated by the heights of the rectangles.

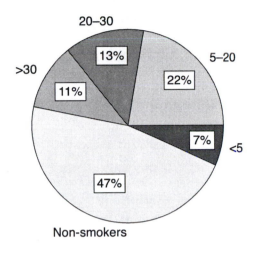

Figure 1.9 Pie-chart – indicating percentages of nurses in a particular institution with regard to their smoking habits.

Two basic types of measure

There are two basic types of measure with which we concern ourselves in dealing with largish samples. Let us consider what they must be by looking at two examples. In out first example, a group of 50 males is tested for blood pH. The 50 are selected as a random sample from a block of flats in East London. In that sample, the mean pH is 7.4, with the lowest reading being 7.0 and the highest reading being 7.8. The *mean*, by the way, simply means adding up all the scores and dividing by the number of scores. There are some interesting features about those figures, but we shall return to them later. We will now consider our second example. Again, we have 50 males and again we measure the blood pH of each. In this case though, they are all Baptist ministers, competing in track and field events at a temperance conference weekend. Their mean pH likewise, is 7.4, but the *range* of obtained readings is much more restricted – 7.35 to 7.46.

It would help if we roughly sketched these two results, as in Figures 10a and 10b. The figures illustrated that it is convenient to have some kind of measure of *central tendency*. In this case, we used the mean, but as we shall see later, there are other measures. The measure of central tendency is a number that we can think of as, in a rough and ready sort of way, representing the whole group. Now, both samples were of males, both samples were of the same size (50) and both had the same mean. But can

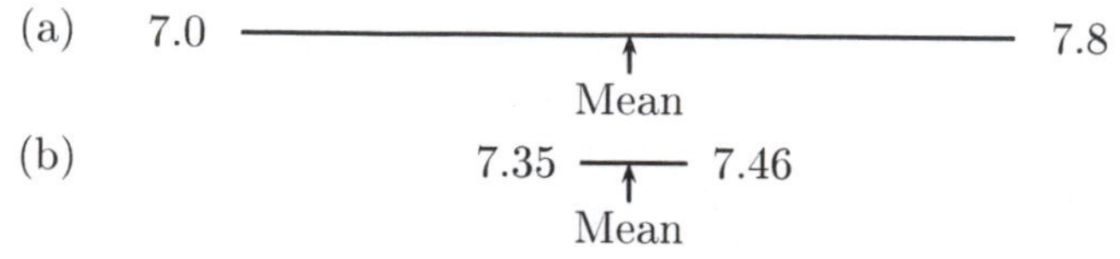

(a)   7.0 ——————————————————— 7.8
                              ↑
                            Mean

(b)   7.35 ——↑—— 7.46
                            Mean

Figure 10 Blood pH readings for 50 males.
(a) East London male sample, (b) Baptist minister male sample.

the two samples be regarded as the same, or even as similar? What differentiates them? Clearly, they are different, and the glaring difference is in the spread of scores. The East London sample could have been made up of males of any age, in any state of health. More to the point, those who were old enough (and maybe even some of those who weren't!) might easily have included drinkers. Among those drinkers, some could have been heavy drinkers. Thus, their blood pHs would vary widely. There might have been only one with a blood pH as low as 6.5 (from really excessive and recent drinking) and 3 or 4 with blood pHs of 7.3 due to illness. In the other sample, the males would all be adult (in order to already be ordained ministers); they would all be teetotallers (because they were Baptist and at a temperance conference), and all reasonably fit (or they wouldn't have entered the track and field events). We would assume of such a sample that, not only would its mean blood pH be normal, but that each one would have a blood pH either normal or very close to it.

In other words, to describe data like this, you need two basic measures:

- a measure of central tendency
- a measure of dispersion (or scatter, or range).

Just as the mean is not the only measure of central tendency, the range is not the only measure of dispersion. The 'mean' (or 'arithmetic mean'), by the way, is simply what we in primary school called the 'average'. Namely, add up all the scores and divide by the number of scores. But in proper statistical parlance an 'average' can be any measure of central tendency, such as a mode or a median.

Measures of central tendency

Other widely-used measures of central tendency are: the *mode* and the *median*. The mode is the score (or measure or datum) occuring most frequently. For instance, among army recruits in a particular country, the authorities might have found that the great majority of soldiers can wear a hat size 7. Some soldiers might find a $7\frac{1}{2}$ more comfortable and some a $6\frac{1}{2}$, but these latter two categories are small in number. In mass-producing the army hats, they would use the mode (hat size 7), knowing that a few would have grossly ill-fitting hats, but that most of the army would be all right! If they used the mean, they could get a figure like 6.9, which fitted no one properly!

The median is that score above (and below) which 50% of the other scores fall. Here is an example which nicely illustrates its use as a measure of central tendency. There are two factories, A and B. Each has the same number of workers, including management. In factory A, the mean salary is £160 per week. In factory B, the mean salary is £140 per week. In which factory would you rather work, given that job satisfaction was otherwise equal in both places?

If you had any sense, you would say: 'I need more information to make an informed choice'. But, if you were bamboozled by the means, you might say, 'factory A, please'. In you go, sunshine! Once there, you find that everyone gets £100 per week, except the boss – and he gets £4000 per week! Oh well, how are things in factory B? In factory B, the range of salaries is £135–£145 per week. The median – the salary below which 50% of the employees get and above which 50% get – is £143 per week. In factory A, the median salary is of course, £100 per week. The boss is just one more earner there and the fact that he pulls down £4000 per week still only puts him among the 50% earning above £100 per week.

From this example, you can see two things.

1   The mean is subject to distortion by extreme values. In factory A, the boss's exorbitant wage raised the mean drastically. Neither the median nor the mode are affected by extreme values.
2   The mean could easily be a measure that is not represented by any actual score in the sample from which it was calculated.

Measures of dispersion

The range is one rough and ready measure of dispersion. To help us consider some others, let us consider a small set of scores

$$4, 4, 5, 6, 7, 7, 7, 7, 9, 9, 10, 16, 16, 16, 17, 18, 18, 19, 19, 24$$

How much does each score (we designate any of the scores as x) deviate from its mean? Well, to find out, we have to first calculate the mean, $\bar{x}$, which is 11.9. (Add all the scores and divide by 20.) So the first score, 4, deviates negatively by 7.9 from the mean, and so on, until we get to the last score, 24, which deviates positively by 12.1 from the mean. In each case, of course, the required calculation is: $x - \bar{x}$. You don't have to be Albert Einstein to appreciate that if the mean had been properly calculated in the first place, the deviations – negative and positive – would cancel each other out. Thus, the idea of simply working out the 'average deviation' as a measure of dispersion would not work. As soon as you added up the deviations to work out their mean the sum would always come to zero!

We can get around this wrinkle by treating each deviation as an absolute value – meaning it has no sign. Absolute values are indicated by a pair of short vertical lines. Thus

$$|x - \bar{x}|$$

means 'the absolute value of $x - \bar{x}$'.

If we add up all the $|x - \bar{x}|$ values, a procedure symbolised by

$$\Sigma|x - \bar{x}|$$

because Σ (or 'sigma') just means 'sum up' or 'add up', we can then easily calculate the mean of the absolute deviations, or *MAD*.

$$MAD = \frac{\Sigma|x - \bar{x}|}{n} = \frac{111}{20} = 5.55$$

That would certainly qualify as a measure of dispersion, but for various mathematical reasons having to do with integral calculus and areas under curves, it is not nearly as useful or as widely used as another measure called the *standard deviation*. Each squared deviation is, of course, a positive number because even if the original deviation had been negative, the square of a negative number is positive. You then take the mean of all the squared deviations

$$\frac{\Sigma(x - \bar{x})^2}{n}$$

This, in itself, is certainly a measure of dispersion, and we call it the *variance*. To get the standard deviation, called σ or 'sigma'*, we simply take the square root of the variance

---

* Sigma: Σ is the capital of this Greek letter and σ is the lower case form of the same Greek letter.

$$\sigma = \sqrt{\frac{\Sigma(x - \bar{x})^2}{n}}$$

Now, we said at the outset that we almost never have access to the whole population of scores, but only a sample. For mathematical reasons beyond the scope of this presentation, the standard deviation of a sample, indicated by sd, is given by

$$sd = \sqrt{\frac{\Sigma(x - \bar{x})^2}{n - 1}}$$

That is, we divide by $(n - 1)$ instead of n. The relevant calculations on this data follow.

In statistics, the measure of central tendency and of dispersion are called 'parameters'. The two basic parameters in statistical calculations are the arithmetic mean and the standard deviation.

Why divide by (n–1) instead of by n?

In order to calculate the mean of, say, 7 numbers, we add them all up and divide by 7. Suppose you knew the mean of the 7 values already, but did not know all the individual values. In that event, how many (as a minimum) of the 7 values must you know in order for the yet unknown one, or ones, to be definitely ascertainable?

For instance, suppose I told you that I have 7 values, the mean of which is 6. What must the values be? Well, you can appreciate that such a question is not answerable with certainty. Obviously, you would have no difficulty in sitting down and finding 7 numbers that the mean of which is 6, but there are many such sets. If your questioner has a particular set in mind, you cannot arrive at a method – on the basis of only knowing the mean – of definitely saying which 7 numbers went into the calculation. All you know is that the seven values must add up to 42, because

$$\frac{\Sigma x}{7} = 6$$

so

$$\Sigma x = 42$$

but all sorts of sets of 7 numbers add up to 42.

Suppose that you were told that one of the values was 5. Would that enable you to find the other 6 values of x?

$$5 + \Sigma x = 42$$

so

$$\Sigma x = 37$$

Again, you are stuck with a similar problem, except that this time you have to find 6 numbers which add up to 37.

You now appreciate, I am sure, that knowing two values for sure (say 5 and 7) would not help. In that case, $\Sigma x = 30$ – but which 5 values can you pick? Likewise, knowing 3 values, say, 5, 7 and 9, still leaves you with having to find a particular 4 numbers which add up to 21. Knowing 4 values, say, 5, 7, 9 and 8, leaves you with the problem of exactly which 3 numbers add up to make 13. Knowing 5 values, say, 5, 7, 9, 8 and 6, leaves you with the problem of stating definitely which 2 numbers add up to 7. It still cannot be done, can it?

Only if you know all but one of the values, and the mean itself, of a set of numbers, can you work out the remaining number. That is, if you have 7 numbers, the first 6 of which are 5, 7, 9, 8, 6 and 4, can you definitely work out the missing one so that their mean is 6?

$$\frac{5 + 7 + 9 + 8 + 6 + 4 + x}{7} = 6$$

$$39 + x = 42$$

so

$$x = 3$$

What this means, in the larger mathematical context, is that in calculating the mean you have lost one 'degree of freedom' – that is, one value remains strictly determined.

Now let us rearrange the data from the beginning of the section. Displayed like this, it is called 'ungrouped data'. We are treating each score individually. This allows perfect accuracy in calculating such parameters as the mean or the standard deviation, but – as you shall soon appreciate – it becomes far too tedious. We get around this by arranging our data as 'grouped data'. For now, though, consider the ungrouped data below.

x	$x - \bar{x}$	$(x - \bar{x})^2$
4	−7.9	62.41
4	−7.9	62.41
5	−6.9	47.61
6	−5.9	34.81
7	−4.9	24.01
7	−4.9	24.01
7	−4.9	24.01
7	−4.9	24.01
9	−2.9	8.41
9	−2.9	8.41
10	−1.9	3.61
16	4.1	16.81
16	4.1	16.81
16	4.1	16.81
17	5.1	26.01
18	6.1	37.21
18	6.1	37.21
19	7.1	50.41
19	7.1	50.41
24	12.1	146.41
$\Sigma x = 238$	$\Sigma\lvert x - \bar{x}\rvert = 111.0$	$\Sigma(x - \bar{x})^2 = 721.80$

mean:

$$\bar{x} = \frac{\Sigma x}{n} = \frac{238}{20} = 11.9$$

mean of absolute deviations:

$$MAD = \frac{\Sigma\lvert x - \bar{x}\rvert}{n} = \frac{111}{20} = 5.55$$

standard deviation:

$$sd = \sqrt{\frac{\Sigma(x - \bar{x})^2}{n - 1}} = \sqrt{\frac{721.80}{19}} = 6.1636$$

Grouped data

Only on fairly small samples can we hope to consider the frequency of each score and work with data on an individual score basis. Even if you have as few as 100 scores, it becomes easier to group the data.

Grouped data is data that involves so many figues that it is set out in class intervals, showing the number of each measure (frequency) that occurs in each interval. A good example, showing the figures for weight loss for 90 people, follows. First, the raw data is presented below.

18.6	13.8	10.4	15.0	16.0	22.1	16.2	36.1	11.6	7.8
22.6	17.9	25.3	32.8	16.6	13.6	8.5	23.7	14.2	22.9
17.7	26.3	9.2	24.9	17.9	26.5	26.6	16.5	18.1	24.8
16.6	32.3	14.0	11.6	20.0	33.8	15.8	15.2	24.0	16.4
24.1	23.2	17.3	10.5	15.0	20.2	20.2	17.3	16.6	16.9
22.0	23.9	24.0	12.2	21.8	12.2	22.0	9.6	8.0	20.4
17.2	18.3	13.0	10.6	17.2	8.9	16.8	14.2	15.7	8.0
17.7	16.1	17.8	11.6	10.4	13.6	8.4	12.6	8.1	11.6
21.1	20.5	19.8	24.8	9.7	25.1	31.8	24.9	20.0	17.6

We shall now 'group' the data to make it more compact. The following table shows how we begin to go about this. The advantages of having groups are obvious. For one thing, it makes it more compact and you get an idea at a quick glance of what its tendencies are. Of course, we have to evolve different formulae for the measure of central tendency and for the measures of dispersion, using grouped data rather than individual measures, but this is quite easily done.

In the table below, notice how we work out the frequency in each interval. As we read out each measure from the raw data, which itself does not have to be listed in ascending order, we put a tally mark (usually a I) opposite the appropriate class interval. We might eventually end up with IIII opposite some interval and then read out another measure that belongs in that interval. We put the fifth tally mark as HH. This makes it easy to read the tally marks in bunches of 5 later on when we are converting them to frequency numbers.

Class boundaries (gm)	Class midpoints (x)	Tallied frequency	Frequency (f)	Cumulative frequency
7.5–10.5	9	HH HH II	12	12
10.5–13.5	12	HH HH	10	22
13.5–16.5	15	HH HH HH	15	37
16.5–19.5	18	HH HH HH IIII	19	56
19.5–22.5	21	HH HH II	12	68
22.5–25.5	24	HH HH IIII	14	82
25.5–28.5	27	IIII	3	85
28.5–31.5	30		0	85
31.5–34.5	33	IIII	4	89
34.5–37.5	36	I	1	90

Notice that we first establish the *class intervals*. These are 7.5–10.5 gm, 10.5–13.5 gm, etc. The midpoints of these intervals are then listed in the next column. We call these midpoints '*x*', because in grouped data each score in any one interval is counted as equal to the midpoint of that interval. Be sure you understand this. Suppose you had an interval 40.5–43.5 and 6 scores fell in that interval, say

$$40.6, 41.3, 41.8, 42.9, 43.1 \text{ and } 43.4$$

We could count each of these scores as '42', the midpoint of 40.5–43.5. This introduces a slight inaccuracy, because the sum of the real scores is 253.1. Using the midpoints, $6 \times 42 = 252$.

But you can appreciate that sometimes your approximation of $f \times x$, or fx, where *x* is the midpoint, will be more than and sometimes less than and sometimes (but rarely) equal to the real value; but with a large number of data, this will roughly balance out. In return for slightly less accurate analysis, we get the convenience which grouped data offers. You may think that with only 90 data, it it not worth the trouble. But health data characteristically involves much more than 90 scores!

You should be able to see that there are certain rules of thumb to be followed, but they are largely common sense. The rules are:

1 The right endpoint (also called *class limit* or *class boundary*) of one class interval is the same as the left endpoint of the next one.
2 We usually design the intervals so that the midpoints are whole numbers rather than fractions.
3 For most data, no fewer than 10 and no more than 20 class intervals are desirable. Fewer than 10 results in too much loss of accuracy, while more than 20 makes it too unwieldy.
4 That means that the class interval should be between $\frac{1}{10}$ and $\frac{1}{20}$ of the difference between the largest and smallest score. (Note that statisticians usually call their measures 'scores'.) In the above example, the difference between the largest and the smallest score is: $36.1 - 7.8 = 28.3$. So for 10 classes some convenient number in the vicinity of 2.82 should be used as the class interval. We shall use class intervals of size 3. Since the first interval has to contain 7.8, we chose 7.5 as the lowest class boundary.

To appreciate how it all works out, look at table below, in which four columns, for $|x - m|, f|x - m|, (x - m)^2$, and $f(x - m)^2$, have been added to facilitate calculation of the parameters.

Class boundaries	x	f	$\lvert x - m \rvert$	$f\lvert x - m \rvert$	$(x - m)^2$	$f(x - m)^2$
7.5–10.5	9	12	9.13	109.56	83.3569	1000.2828
10.5–13.5	12	10	6.13	61.30	37.5769	375.7690
13.5–16.5	15	15	3.13	46.95	9.7969	146.9535
16.5–19.5	18	19	0.13	2.47	0.0169	0.3211
19.5–22.5	21	12	2.87	34.44	8.2369	98.8428
22.5–25.5	24	14	5.87	82.18	34.4596	482.3965
25.5–28.5	27	3	8.87	26.61	78.6769	236.0307
28.5–31.5	30	0	11.87	0.00	140.8969	0.0000
31.5–34.5	33	4	14.87	59.48	221.1169	884.4676
34.5–37.5	36	1	17.87	17.87	319.3369	319.3369
				440.86		3544.4009

We leave this data for a few moments to explain a few elementary things about calculating with grouped data.

Calculating with grouped data

Common sense comes to our rescue here. The reason for grouping the data in the first place is to avoid having to work tediously with individual scores. If you give a first aid test to 20 people and end up with the following list of scores:

$$83, 83, 83, 83, 88, 88, 90, 90, 90, 90, 90, 90, 90, 94, 94, 94, 98, 100, 100, 100$$

you could calculate the mean by adding them up and dividing by 20. But it would make a lot more sense to do it as follows

$$\bar{x} = \frac{4 \times 83 + 2 \times 88 + 7 \times 90 + 3 \times 94 + 1 \times 98 + 3 \times 100}{20}$$

That is, if f_i is the frequency with which the score x_i occured, then your formula would be

$$\frac{\sum_{N}^{i=1} f_i x_i}{total}$$

where N is the number of *clusters* and not the total number of scores. The total number of scores should be the sum of the frequencies

$$\sum_{N}^{i=1} f_i = 4 + 2 + 7 + 3 + 1 + 3 = 20$$

If it isn't, you've done something wrong. So, our formula for the mean would be

$$\bar{x} = \frac{\sum_{N}^{i=1} f_i x_i}{\sum_{N}^{i=1} f_i}$$

Now with grouped data, we follow the common sense approach precisely, using the midpoints of the interval as our scores. If m stands for mean and x stands for score, the $|x - m|$ is the absolute value of the difference between a score and the mean. I have deliberately used m instead of $\bar{x}$ for mean, and x instead of x_i for score, because you will find differences like that as you move from one person's statistics to another's. The symbols are not as well-established as they are in other branches of mathematics.

I now calculate, for each interval, $|x - m|$ (which I will need if I want to calculate the mean deviation), $|x - m| \times f$ (meaning the frequency times each deviation – to calculate the mean deviation), $(x - m)^2$ (to calculate the standard deviation and variance), and $(x - m)^2 f$ (meaning frequency times each square of deviation – to calculate the mean deviation).

Returning to our grouped data

Now you should have no difficulty understanding the following calculations. Remember, you will never have to do such calculations as the computer programme will do it for you. But be sure that you understand it. It will allow you to use your computer results with much more intelligence and confidence.

You have already seen that in grouped data

mean:

$$m = \frac{\Sigma f_i x_i}{\Sigma f_i}$$

mean deviation:

$$md = \frac{\Sigma f |x_i - m|}{\Sigma f_i}$$

standard deviation:

$$sd = \sqrt{\frac{\Sigma f (x_i - m)^2}{\Sigma f_i}}$$

variance:

$$var = (sd)^2$$

So in the grouped data we have been given

$$sd = \sqrt{\frac{3544.4009}{90}} = \sqrt{39.38} = 6.28g$$

The mode is no problem. Just pick the class interval with the highest frequency. In our data, the mode is the interval 16.5g–19.5g, represented by the midpoint 18g. The only really tricky thing to calculate from grouped data is the median. There are 90 scores, so we have to find a score below which 45 scores fall and above which 45 scores fall. Let us start adding up the frequencies, starting with the lowest class interval, until we get to 45. $12 + 10 = 22, 22 + 15 = 37, 37 + 19 = 56$ – oops! We've passed it. What do we do?

Well, we know that the median is in the interval (16.5–19.5) somewhere, because below that interval fall 37 scores, and its own scores bring the total past 45. We are going to have to work it out by proportion.

It is going to be 16.5 plus something. Up to 16.5 we have 37 scores. We need 8 more scores to get up to 45. But there are 19 scores in that interval. So we need $\frac{8}{19}$ of that interval – right! The interval is 3, so we calculate

$$\frac{8}{19} \times 3 = \frac{24}{19} \approx 1.2$$

Therefore, our median is about $16.5 + 1.2 = 17.7$.

An alternative formula for the standard deviation

You may think that you need this like a hole in the head, but it is going to come in useful in Chapter 6. We are going to prove that

$$\sqrt{\frac{\Sigma(x - \bar{x})^2}{n - 1}} = \sqrt{\frac{\Sigma x^2 - \frac{(\Sigma x)^2}{n}}{n - 1}}$$

Unless you are interested and just do not like to accept things on my say-so, you don't need to deal with this algebraic proof. But for the interested here it is.

I'll start you off on one way to go about it, although there is more than one way of divesting a domestic feline of its integumentary covering. Start off with expanding $(x - \bar{x})^2$, so we get

$$\frac{\Sigma(x - \bar{x})^2}{n - 1} = \frac{\Sigma x^2 - \Sigma 2x\bar{x} + \Sigma\bar{x}^2}{n - 1}$$

OK, now, 2 is a constant and so is $\bar{x}$ (once it is calculated), so $2\bar{x}$ can come out to the other side of the Σ sign in the middle term

$$\frac{\Sigma(x - \bar{x})^2}{n - 1} = \frac{\Sigma x^2 - 2\bar{x}\Sigma x + \Sigma\bar{x}^2}{n - 1}$$

$$= \frac{\Sigma x^2 - \dfrac{2\Sigma x}{n}\Sigma x + n(\bar{x})^2}{n - 1}$$

If you cannot see that $\Sigma\bar{x}^2 = n(\bar{x})^2$, think of it this way: $\bar{x}$ is a constant, unlike x itself. Suppose you wanted to add

$$15^2 + 15^2 + 15^2 + 15^2 + 15^2 + 15^2 + 15^2$$

You could write $\sum 15^2$, but then you could also write 7×15^2.

OK, back to the salt mine

$$\frac{\Sigma(x - x)^2}{n - 1} = \frac{\Sigma x^2 - \dfrac{2\Sigma x^2}{n} + n\left(\dfrac{\Sigma x^2}{n^2}\right)}{n - 1}$$

$$= \frac{\Sigma x^2 - \dfrac{2\Sigma x^2}{n} + \dfrac{\Sigma x^2}{n}}{n - 1}$$

$$= \frac{\Sigma x^2 - \dfrac{(\Sigma x)^2}{n}}{n - 1}$$

Home and hosed!

$$\sqrt{\frac{(x - \bar{x})^2}{n - 1}}$$

and

$$\sqrt{\frac{\Sigma x^2 - \dfrac{(\Sigma x)^2}{n}}{n-1}}$$

are both expressions for the standard deviation of x. I didn't need to do the whole thing for you, but I'm soft-hearted.

Which formula do you use? It makes no difference. Use the one that most conveniently fits the way your data is presented. But I think you can see that the first formula involves calculating each deviation and then squaring each deviation. The second formula does not require either of these tedious calculations!

Study exercises

Periodically throughout the book, I set some simple problems just to help the reader make sure that the material is being understood. In most cases, the answers are provided – but not always! In the problems that follow, a calculator would save you a lot of bother. Also, you may need reminding of what we mean by 'two decimal places of accuracy'. It means, calculate the answers to have three decimal places (three digits to the right of the decimal point). For instance, suppose your calculator gives you a mean of 7.018743. Retain only 7.018. Now to get two decimal places of accuracy, look at the third digit to the right of the decimal point. If it is 5 or more, raise the second digit to the right of the decimal point by 1. So 7.018 would be 7.02 to two decimal places of accuracy. Otherwise, do not raise the second digit to the right of the decimal point. So, 15.42499 would be 15.42 to two decimal places of accuracy.

Study exercises 1

You need a lot of practice now and here it is. I hope you have a calculator!

1 For the set of numbers 6.5, 8.3, 4.7, 9.2, 11.3, 8.5, 9.5, 9.2, calculate to two decimal places:
   (a) the mean
   (b) the median
   (c) the mean deviation
   (d) the standard deviation.

2   Given the following frequency distribution:

Class boundary	Frequency
10–30	5
30–50	8
50–70	12
70–90	18
90–110	3
110–130	2

Find to two decimal places:
(a) the mean
(b) the median
(c) the modal class
(d) the mean deviation
(e) the standard deviation, using the definition.

3   Measurements of lengths, in cm, of 50 EKG strips are distributed as follows:

Class boundary	Frequency
2.35–2.45	1
2.45–2.55	4
2.55–2.65	7
2.65–2.75	15
2.75–2.85	11
2.85–2.95	10
2.95–3.05	2

Find to two decimal places:
(a) the mean
(b) the median
(c) the modal class
(d) the mean deviation
(e) the standard deviation, using the definition.

Chapter 2

A necessary glimpse of probability

The problem of statistical inference

In ordinary parlance, two broad categories of statistics are recognised – *descriptive* statistics and *inferential* statistics. Descriptive statistics includes all of the techniques used to present data and to discuss its general configuration. For instance, graphs, histograms, frequency polygons, etc., are all part of descriptive statistics, as are also the measures of central tendency and of dispersion – the parameters, as statisticians call them.

Inferential statistics, on the other hand, concerns itself with drawing inferences of a probabilistic nature from a given description of data. For instance, it might be said that, from analysis of a particular set of scores representing the heights of a group of men, that the probability of someone being 180 cm tall or more is 0.15. Obviously, inferential statistics is a vital branch of the subject, for it is all that gives life and meaning and utility to the whole enterprise. However, in order to make such inferences, or to understand them when they are made by others, one must have a basic grasp of how the mathematics of probability works. This is a difficult undertaking for people who are not mathematically inclined, because it is one of those topics which seems so ambiguous and imprecise. This is only an impression, though. Actually, probability theory is as definite and as rigorous as any other branch of mathematics.

In this chapter, I have attempted to explain those rudiments of it which you will need to think effectively about inferential statistics and to use important statistical tests. To simplify things, we start off with such phenomena as coin throws, dice, draws of cards, etc. These phenomena are strictly limited in range and character and thus can be described exhaustively. By making analogies with these simple situations, we can then go on to the more abstract realm of medical statistical inference. However, this will only work if you thoroughly understand all of the less esoteric phenomena associated with coins, dice and cards.

Some basic laws of probability

Probability laws are useful for faster calculation of probabilities. The first of these laws requires the following definition.

If two or more events are such that not more than one of them can occur in a single trial, they are said to be *mutually exclusive.*

In a single draw from a deck of playing cards the two events of obtaining an ace and obtaining a king are mutually exclusive, whereas the two events of drawing an ace and drawing a spade are not mutually exclusive, since in a particular draw a card may be both an ace and a spade.

If p_1, p_2, p_3, . . . , p_r are the separate probabilites of the occurrence of r mutually exclusive events, the probability P that any one of these events will occur in a single trial is

$$P = p_1 + p_2 + p_3 + ... + p_r$$

An example will help to make this clear. Find the probability of drawing an ace, king, or queen from a regular 4-suit, 52-card deck of cards. The probability p_1 of drawing an ace in a single trial is $\frac{4}{52} = \frac{1}{13}$; the probability p_2 of drawing a king is $\frac{1}{13}$; and the probability of drawing a queen is $\frac{1}{13}$. Since these events are mutually exclusive, the probability of drawing an ace, or a king or a queen is

$$P = \frac{1}{13} + \frac{1}{13} + \frac{1}{13} = \frac{3}{13}$$

which could also have been found directly from the definition of probability.

Of course, this says nothing about events which are *not* mutually exclusive. Two or more events are said to be *independent* if the probability of the occurrence of one of them is not influenced by the occurrence of the other. For instance, the probability that you will get out of bed in the morning is dependent on the probability that you will go to bed the night before. But the probability that you will get out of bed in the morning is independent of the probability that later on that day you will get a telephone bill!

With mutually exclusive events, we are usually interested in the probability of one or the other. With independent events we are usually concerned with the probability of one occurring and the other occurring. For instance, if the probability of throwing a 4 or a 5 in dice is $\frac{2}{6}$ (work it out) and the probability of drawing a king out of a deck of cards is $\frac{1}{13}$ (because $\frac{4}{52} = \frac{1}{13}$), what is the probability that in throwing the dice you get a 4 or a 5 and then in the drawing of a card you get a king? The best way to imagine this is to think of your chances of each successive event being successively reduced. The probability of success in the dice throw is $\frac{1}{3}$. So you are now operating on only $\frac{1}{3}$ of a chance. Within that $\frac{1}{3}$, what is the probability of drawing a king? Well, it has to be $\frac{1}{13}$ of the $\frac{1}{3}$, that is

$$\frac{1}{13} \times \frac{1}{3} = \frac{1}{39}$$

Thus we can say: If $p_1, p_2, p_3, \ldots, p_r$ are the separate probabilities of r independent events, then the probability that all of them will occur in a single trial is given by

$$p_1 p_2 p_3 \cdots p_r$$

Take another example. If the probability of being born blind is $\frac{1}{10}$ and the probability of going deaf is $\frac{1}{4}$, what is the probability of being born blind and going deaf – assuming that these probabilities are independent?

Well there is a probability of $\frac{1}{10}$ of being born blind. If you were not born blind, it wouldn't matter whether you went deaf or not – you would never satisfy the condition of being born blind *and* going deaf. So you have already cut the probability out of which you are operating down to $\frac{1}{10}$. See the pie chart in Figure 2.1. Now, what is the probability that (a) you are within the 'born blind' wedge and *then* go deaf. Well, it must be $\frac{1}{4}$ of that wedge, because whenever you are in the pie diagram you have a $\frac{1}{4}$ chance of going deaf. So, the probability of being born blind *and* going deaf is

$$\frac{1}{10} \times \frac{1}{4} = \frac{1}{40}$$

Here's another example. From a deck of 52 cards a card is withdrawn at random and not replaced. A second card is then drawn. What is the probability that the first card is an ace and the second a king?

Now the probability of getting an ace on the first draw is $\frac{1}{13}$ and of getting a king on the second draw, after an ace has been withdrawn, is $\frac{4}{51}$. Therefore the desired probability is

$$P = \frac{1}{13} \cdot \frac{4}{51} = \frac{4}{663}$$

This means that in the long run of drawing two cards in a row, when the first

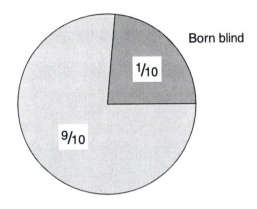

Figure 2.1 Pie chart showing the proportion of people born blind in the example, only the shaded region contributes to the final probability.

card drawn is not replaced, an ace followed by a king will occur only 4 in 663 times or about once in 166 trials.*

Probability in health calculations

The mathematics of probability and the (often unstated) assumptions about it underlie much of what is discussed in public health and epidemiology. A very practical example of this arises in connection with genetics and inherited illnesses, such as haemophilia and sickle cell anaemia. A few simple ideas about probability provide the basis for this.

For instance, if the probability that it will rain tommorrow is $\frac{3}{8}$, then the probability that it won't rain tommorrow is $\frac{5}{8}$. If the probability of you winning the National Lottery main prize is $\frac{1}{14000000}$, then the probability that you won't win is $\frac{13999999}{14000000}$, which, of course, is virtually certain! In a Brent supermarket the author once saw an advertisement for a diet regime which posed the question: 'Do you want to lose 10 pounds fast?' Under which some wag had scrawled: 'Then buy 10 National Lottery tickets'.

---

*Note that a dot placed in the midline position between two quantities in mathematics indicates multiplication.

The point is that, with respect to any one event, all the probabilities must add up to one. In our above examples

$$\frac{3}{8} + \frac{5}{8} = \frac{8}{8} = 1$$

and

$$\frac{1}{14000000} + \frac{13999999}{14000000} = \frac{14000000}{14000000} = 1$$

Applying this to the probability of inheriting a genetic illness, let us suppose that the probability of inheriting the illness is $\frac{1}{8}$, then the probability of not inheriting it is $\frac{7}{8}$. If the parents know this, they can calculate the probabilities for different numbers of children as follows. Let p be the probability that the event happens and q be the probability that it doesn't. Then

$$p + q = 1$$

Suppose you have three children. Then we calculate

$$(p + q)^3$$

Be sure that you remember what the little '3' means. It means 'cubed' or the 'power of three'. In case you are a bit rusty about this, read the following carefully:

4^3 means $4 \times 4 \times 4$ or 64

2^7 means $2 \times 2 \times 2 \times 2 \times 2 \times 2 \times 2$ or 128 (work it out).

And now another question is sure to arise, because it has every time I teach this topic to public health researchers. The question is: If we want to know the probabilities for illness among three children, there are four possible scenarios:

1   All three have the illness. From what we have done before, you can see that this would be

$$\frac{1}{8} \times \frac{1}{8} \times \frac{1}{8} = \left(\frac{1}{8}\right)^3 = \frac{1}{512}$$

2   But you could have two with the condition and one without it

$$\left(\frac{1}{8}\right)^2 \times \left(\frac{7}{8}\right) = \frac{7}{512}$$

3   Or you could have only one with the condition and two without it

$$\left(\frac{1}{8}\right) \times \left(\frac{7}{8}\right)^2 = \frac{49}{512}$$

4   Or, by very good luck, you could have three children without the condition

$$\left(\frac{7}{8}\right)^3 = \frac{343}{512}$$

That is, each child (in this context) is an *event* in the complete *probability* space. The probability space is the list of all possible outcomes (as shown from 1 to 4 above) for that situation.

Now each of those four events is not equally likely. If you read on, you will see how we work out what the probabilities of each of three events is. But first, how do we raise $(p+q)$ to some power. Well, $(p+q)^1$ is simply $(p+q)$, so if you have only one child, the chance that it will have the disease is p. If the p happens to be $\frac{1}{8}$, then the probability that the baby will inherit the illness is $\frac{1}{8}$. Suppose you have two children. Then you must calculate $(p+q)^2$

$$(p+q)^2 = (p+q)(p+q)$$

But

$$(p+q)(p+q) = p(p+q) + q(p+q)$$

$$= p^2 + pq + qp + q^2$$

so $(p+q)^2 = p^2 + 2pq + q^2$ (because $pq = qp$).

Thus our probability space shows that there are three possibilities and gives the probabilities of each. So our probability space is as follows.

1   Both children have the condition. The probability of that is p^2. If $p = \frac{1}{8}$, that gives $\frac{1}{64}$.
2   One child has the condition and one does not. That turns out to have a probability of $2pq$, or $2 \times \frac{1}{8} \times \frac{7}{8}$, which is $\frac{14}{64}$.

3 The only other possibility in this probability space is that both children do not have the condition. That is q^2 or $(\frac{7}{8})^2$, which is $\frac{49}{64}$.

Add up these probabilities and they come to one. If your probability space does not add up to one, you have made a mistake.

$$\frac{1}{64} + \frac{14}{64} + \frac{49}{64} = 1$$

Binomials raised to various powers

Reminding the reader of a bit of elementary algebra, any algebraic expression like $(p + q)$, that involves adding (or subtracting) two different terms is called a *binomial*. So when we deal with inherited illness, a lot of our calculations will involve raising the binomial $(p + q)$ to different powers. In algebra, this is called, naturally enough, 'binomial expansion'. Hence, let us get a bit of practice with binomial expansions.

We already know that

$$(p + q)^2 = p^2 + 2pq + q^2$$

So

$$
\begin{aligned}
(p + q)^3 &= (p + q)(p^2 + 2pq + q^2) \\
&= p(p^2 + 2pq + q^2) + q(p^2 + 2pq + q^2) \\
&= p^3 + 2p^2q + pq^2 + qp^2 + 2pq^2 + q^3 \\
&= p^3 + 3p^2q + 3pq^2 + q^3
\end{aligned}
$$

Be careful with what can and cannot be added together. $2p^2q$ can be added to qp^2 because qp^2 is the same as p^2q, so $2p^2q + qp^2 = 3p^2q$. As we say in school, p^2q and qp^2 are 'like terms'. But you cannot add p^2q and pq^2. These are 'unlike terms'. So $2pq^2$ can be added to pq^2 to get $3pq^2$. If you practice it carefully, you will see that

$$
\begin{aligned}
(p + q)^4 &= (p + q)(p^3 + 3p^2q + 3pq^2 + q^3) \\
&= p(p^3 + 3p^2q + 3pq^2 + q^3) + q(p^3 + 3p^2q + 3pq^2 + q^3) \\
&= p^4 + 4p^3q + 6p^2q^2 + 4pq^3 + q^4
\end{aligned}
$$

Similarly

$$(p+q)^5 = p^5 + 5p^4q + 10p^3q^2 + 10p^2q^3 + 5pq^4 + q^4$$

That is enough! Let us now look for a pattern that will enable you to do such binomial expansions without having to do all of that gory algebra.

Take $(p+q)^5$. The first term of the expansion is p^5. The second term has p^4q (for now we will leave out the number in front of each different term – these numbers, by the way, are called coefficients in algebra). So the different terms in the expansion of $(p+q)^5$ are

$$p^5, p^4q, p^3q^2, p^2q^3, pq^4, q^5$$

What do you notice? Well, if a letter has no power written, remember the power is 1. So $p^4q = p^4q^1$. Writing the unlike terms out again, with this in mind we have

$$p^5, p^4q^1, p^3q^2, p^2q^3, p^1q^4, q^5$$

See the pattern? In successive unlike terms in the expansion, the power of p drops 1 and the power of q gains 1. Just to be sure that you understand, try to write out the sequence of unlike terms of $(p+q)^6$. Do it yourself first without looking further at this page! You should have got

$$p^6, p^5q^1, p^4q^2, p^3q^3, p^2q^4, p^1q^5, q^6$$

If you didn't get that, it would be worth your while to go over your work again until you get it right.

Now, the pattern shows us something else. The sums of the powers in each term comes to six.

$$6+0 = 6, 5+1 = 6, 4+2 = 6, 3+3 = 6, 2+4 = 6, 1+5 = 6, 0+6 = 6.$$

Cunning! Try $(p+q)^7$. You should get

$$p^7, p^6q^1, p^5q^2, p^4q^3, p^3q^4, p^2q^5, p^1q^6, q^7$$

But there is a further treat in store! You can now learn a simple way of working out the coefficients. Let us do it on $(p+q)^5$ because we already know the coefficients

$$(p+q)^5 = p^5 + 5p^4q^1 + 10p^3q^2 + 10p^2q^3 + 5p^1q^4 + q^5$$

$$= 1p^5 + 5p^4q^1 + 10p^3q^2 + 10p^2q^3 + 5p^1q^4 + 1q^5$$

The coefficient of the first term is always going to be one, so we just need to calculate the coefficients of the second, third, fourth, fifth and sixth term. Notice, by the way, that if the power of the binomial is two, there are three terms. If the power is three, there are four terms. If the power is four there are five terms and if the power is five there are six terms. If the power of the binomial is six, there are seven terms, etc. This of course, corresponds to the number of possibilities in the probability space.

We are looking at the expansion of $(p+q)^5$

$$(p+q)^5 = 1p^5 + 5p^4q^1 + 10p^3q^2 + 10p^2q^3 + 5p^1q^4 + 1q^5$$

Look at the second term, $5p^4q$. To get the coefficient of the second term we go to the first term. Multiply the power of p by the coefficient of the first term. That gives $5 \times 1 = 5$. Now divide by the number of terms you already have. Well, you only have the first term, $5/1 = 1$. So the coefficient of the second term will be 5.

OK, now let us work out the coefficient of the third term. To do that, we go to the second term, $5p^4q^1$. Multiply the power of p (which is 4) by the coefficient of that term (which is 5), $4 \times 5 = 20$. Now divide 20 by the number of terms you have already done (which is 2). $20 \div 2 = 10$. So the coefficient of the third term is 10.

It should now be easy. To get the coefficient of the fourth term, we look at the third term, $10p^3q^2$. $3 \times 10 = 30$, divided by 3 (because you have done 3 terms) and, of course, you get 10 again. To get the coefficient of the fifth term, look at the fourth term, $10p^2q^3$. Well, $2 \times 10 = 20$, divided by 4 is 5. So the coefficient of the fifth term is 5. You can even work out the coefficient of the sixth term, even though you already know it is 1. Take the fifth term, $5p^1q^4$. $1 \times 5 = 5$. $5 \div 5 = 1$.

Brilliant! Now, just to be absolutely sure that you have it, try to expand $(p+q)^6$. Write the seven unlike terms, leaving a space for the coefficient and then, one by one, work out the coefficients. You will quickly discover another useful pattern, which will stand you in good stead if you are working out genetic ratios as a field doctor with no computer to help out

$$(p+q)^6 = p^6 + 6p^5q^1 + 15p^4q^2 + 20p^3q^3 + 15p^2q^4 + 6p^1q^5 + q^6$$

So if a couple have six children, what is the probability (assuming that $p = \frac{1}{8}$ for the particular condition) that they will have four children with the condition and two without. This would correspond to the term with p^4q^2. You can see from the expansion that that term is $15p^4q^2$. This will tell us that the probability of that event taking place is

$$15p^4q^2 = 15 \times \left(\frac{1}{8}\right)^4 \times \left(\frac{7}{8}\right)^2$$

$$= \frac{15 \times 49}{8^4 \times 8^2}$$

$$= \frac{735}{262144}$$

You can see that each of the seven possibilities has a probability with 8^6 (or 262144) in the denominator. You will meet these fascinating ideas again more formally in Chapter 4, when we deal with binomial distributions.

Permutations

A 'permutation' is an 'arrangement' of items or of events, Suppose that you have four glass ornaments of animals: horse (H), dog (D), cat (C) and elephant (E); and that you want to find all the ways (permutations) of arranging them in a row. We could arbitrarily start off with H and D, in that order. But there are only two ways of arranging C and E, namely: CE or EC. So our first two arrangements would be:

HDCE

HDEC

We could now find all of the ways of arranging DCE. They are:

DCE

DEC

CDE

CED

EDC

ECD

That means that there are six ways of arranging them if we begin each arrangement with H, namely:

HDCE
HDEC
HCDE
HCED
HEDC
HECD

Likewise, there are six ways of arranging them if we begin with D:

DHCE
DHEC
DEHC
DECH
DCHE
DCEH

And there are six ways of arranging them if we begin with C:

CHDE
CHED
CEHD
CEDH
CDHE
CDEH

And finally, there are six ways of arranging them if we begin with E:

EHDC
EHCD
EDHC
EDCH
ECHD
ECDH

Thus, the number of permutations of four things is 24. Is there any way of arriving at this by a more mathematical argument? Yes, there is: there are four ways of filling the first choice of glass animal: H, D, C or E. For each of these possible choices of the first animal, there are 3 choices of the second animal. That means that there are 12 (namely 4×3) ways of choosing the first two animals. Now there are only 2 unassigned animals left. The third one can be chosen in two possible ways, making 24 ways of choosing the first three – and, of course, the fourth animal is the one left. Thus there are $4 \times 3 \times 2 \times 1$ permutations of four things.

It is not difficult to see that, if there were seven different things, we could choose the first one in seven ways, we could choose the second one in six ways, and so on, making $7 \times 6 \times 5 \times 4 \times 3 \times 2 \times 1$ permutations of seven things.

Factorial notation

Permutations, and similar phenomena, constitute such an important part in statistical calculations that we have to find a simpler way of recording them. To do this, we use what is known as *factorial notation*. 'Factorial' (meaning multiply from the whole number specified down by ones to one) is indicated by an exclamation mark. Thus 5! means

$$5 \times 4 \times 3 \times 2 \times 1$$

It is vital that you get used to this symbolism and learn to think with it. Thus, what is the value of

$$\frac{7!}{4!}$$

We could find out by expanding both the numerator and denominator and cancelling as required

$$\frac{7!}{4!} = \frac{7 \times 6 \times 5 \times 4 \times 3 \times 2 \times 1}{4 \times 3 \times 2 \times 1}$$

$$= 7 \times 6 \times 5$$

$$= 210$$

Once you begin to 'imagine' with the notation itself, though, you won't need to laboriously put in the intermediate steps. For instance, what is the value of

$$\frac{9!}{5!}$$

? Well

$$\frac{9!}{5!} = 9 \times 8 \times 7 \times 6$$

We don't need to go further than 6, because $5 \times 4 \times 3 \times 2 \times 1$ all cancels with 5! in the denominator.

Zero factorial

Here is another potentially tricky issue. What does 0! equal? Since factorial indicates the number of permutations, the question is: How many ways are there of arranging an empty set? The answer is not 'none', because the existence of such a set is itself an 'arrangement' of it. Equally obviously, there is only the one way of arranging it. Thus $0! = 1$. Also, of course, $1! = 1$ and $2! = 2$, but $3! = 6$, $4! = 24$, etc.

Calculating with permutations

In discussing factorial notation, we have already dealt with permutations. You remember that a permutation is an arrangement. The number of possible permutations of nine things is given by

$$9! = 9 \times 8 \times 7 \times 6 \times 5 \times 4 \times 3 \times 2 \times 1$$

Another way of illustrating permutations is to think of a tree diagram (Figure 2.2). For instance, what are the permutations of the four letters A, B, C and D? If we start with A, our possible choices of second letter are three (B, C or D). If we choose C, our possible choices of third letter are two (B or D). If we then choose B, our choice of fourth letter is only D. So there are six permutations beginning with A. Likewise, there are six permutations beginning with B, six beginning with C and six beginning with D. Therefore, the number of permutations of n things is given by the formula

$$P = n!$$

Suppose though, you had four things, say letters A, B, C and D, and you wanted to know how many arrangements of three of them were possible. Well, that is not too difficult because you have four possible ways of picking the first letter, that leaves you with three possible ways of picking the second

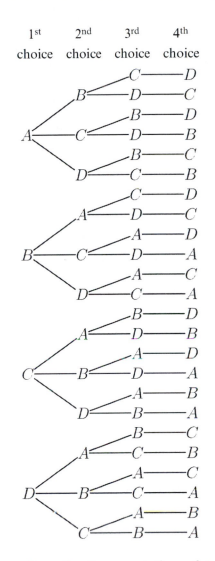

Figure 2.2 Tree diagram illustrating the permutations of A, B, C, D.

letter, that leaves you with two possible ways of picking the third letter – a total of $4 \times 3 \times 2 = 24$ ways.

What is the number of permutations of seven things three at a time? That is, if you have seven things, how many arrangements of three things are there?

Again, you have seven choices for the first thing, six choices for the second thing and five choices for the third thing – a total of

$$7 \times 6 \times 5$$

Put into factorial notation, do you see that this is

$$\frac{7!}{4!}$$

because

$$\frac{7!}{4!} = \frac{7 \times 6 \times 5 \times 4!}{4!}$$

.

Now, we were asked to make arrangements of three things from a choice of seven things. As it turns out. $4 = 7 - 3$, so we could write our answer as

$$\frac{7!}{(7-3)!} = \frac{7!}{4!}$$

$$= 7 \times 6 \times 5$$

So the number of permutations of seven things taken three at a time is given by

$$P_{7,3} = \frac{7!}{(7-3)!}$$

We can generalise that to: the number of permutations of n things taken r at a time is

$$P_{n,r} = \frac{n!}{(n-r)!}$$

Combinations

'Combinations' are more restrictive than 'permutations'. For instance, if we list the 24 permutations of $ABCD$, we get

$ABCD$	$BACD$	$CABD$	$DACB$
$ABDC$	$BADC$	$CADB$	$DABC$
$ACBD$	$BDAC$	$CBAD$	$DCAB$
$ACDB$	$BDCA$	$CBDA$	$DCBA$
$ADBC$	$BCAD$	$CDAB$	$DBAC$
$ADCB$	$BCDA$	$CDBA$	$DBCA$

But out of all of these permutations there is only one combination – because in two different permutations, the same things do not count as different combinations.

If we have five (say *A*, *B*, *C*, *D* and *E*) things taken three at a time, the number of permutations taken three at a time is given by

$$P_{5,3} = \frac{5!}{(5-3)!}$$

But among those permutations, *ABC*, *ACB*, *BCA*, *BAC*, *CBA* and *CAB* will all be counted as separate permutations. Now if we want the number of combinations of five things taken three at a time ($C_{5,3}$) we have to divide the number of permutations ($P_{5,3}$) by 3! because every three different things in $P_{5,3}$ is itself arranged in 3! ways. Since all 3! of these permutations all count as the *same* combination, if we divide $P_{5,3}$ by 3! we will get the number of combinations of five things taken three at a time.

That is, the number of combinations of five things taken three at a time is given by

$$C_{5,3} = \frac{P_{5,3}}{3!} = \frac{5!}{(5-3)!3!}$$

So the number of combinations of *n* things taken *r* at a time must be

$$C_{n,r} = \frac{n!}{r!(n-r)!}$$

The big problem that you will have in doing problems associated with permutations and combinations will involve deciding whether you are dealing with a 'perm' or a 'com'. You can tell which by the wording of the problem. Think in each case: Is it the order of the things in each cluster that counts or is it the number of different clusters? If the order of things in each cluster is important, you are talking about *permutations*. If you are just concerned with the number of clusters, you are dealing with *combinations*.

An example will help. A student body president is asked to appoint a committee consisting of five boys and three girls. He is given a list of ten boys and seven girls from which to make the appointments. From how many possible committees must he make his selection?

He just has to pick five boys from a list of ten boys and three girls from a list of seven girls. The order in which he phones them up and tells them that they have been selected doesn't matter, does it? So we are dealing with combinations.

For the boys, this is

$$C_{10,5} = \frac{10!}{5!(10-5)!} = \frac{10!}{5!5!} = 252$$

For the girls, this is

$$C_{7,3} = \frac{7!}{3!(7-3)!} = \frac{7!}{3!4!} = 35$$

There are 252 ways of picking the boys and 35 ways of picking the girls, so there are

$$252 \times 35 = 8820$$

ways of selecting the committee.

Repeated trials

We can now relate all of this back to probability theory. Suppose in a throw of a dice you want a '3'. The probability of success on a single trial is

$$p = \frac{1}{6}$$

while the probability of failure on a single trial is

$$q = \frac{5}{6}$$

Now, suppose you throw a dice 4 times in a row. You might get

4 successes in a row
3 successes and 1 failure
2 successes and 2 failures
1 success and 3 failures
4 failures in a row.

If you got, say, 1 success and 3 failures, would it make any difference whether your success came first followed by the 3 failures

sfff?

or second: fsff?

or third: ffsf?

or fourth: fffs?

Of course not! So really you need to know the number of ways you can select 3 things out of 4 trials where the order does not count.

$$C_{4,3} = \frac{4!}{1!3!} = 4$$

There are 4 ways that can happen, but out of how many possible outcomes. Well on the first trial you can *succeed* or *fail* (2). The second trial is not influenced by the result of the first trial so on the second trial you can *succeed* or *fail* (2). On the third trial you can *succeed* or *fail* (2). On the fourth trial you can *succeed* or *fail* (2). So there are $2 \times 2 \times 2 \times 2 = 16$ possible outcomes. We have found that 4 of them will give 3 successes and 1 failure.

How many ways are there of getting all successes? That is, how many ways are there of combining 4 things 4 at a time? Only 1 obviously. Even if your common sense does not tell you that, the formula does

$$C_{4,4} = \frac{4!}{0!4!} = 1$$

How many ways of getting 2 successes and 2 failures?

$$C_{4,2} = \frac{4!}{2!2!} = 6$$

How many ways of getting 1 success and 3 failures?

$$C_{4,1} = \frac{4!}{1!3!} = 4$$

How many ways of getting 0 successes and 4 failures?

$$C_{4,0} = \frac{4!}{4!0!} = 1$$

So our 16 possible outcomes of successes/failures in the 4 throws of a dice are:

1	(4 successes)
4	(3 successes, 1 failure)
6	(2 successes, 2 failures)
4	(1 success, 3 failures)
1	(0 successes, 4 failures)
16	

Now we must work out in each single trial what the probability of success or failure is. Well, the probability of success is $p = \frac{1}{6}$ and of failure is $q = \frac{5}{6}$. So the probability of 4 successes is

$$p \times p \times p \times p = p^4 = \left(\frac{1}{6}\right)^4 = \frac{1}{1296}$$

The probability of 3 successes and 1 failures is

$$p \times p \times p \times q = p^3 q = \left(\frac{1}{6}\right)^3 \left(\frac{5}{6}\right) = \frac{5}{1296}$$

The probability of 2 successes and 2 failures is

$$p \times p \times q \times q = p^2 q^2 = \left(\frac{1}{6}\right)^2 \left(\frac{5}{6}\right)^2 = \frac{25}{1296}$$

The probability of 1 success and 3 failures is

$$p \times q \times q \times q = p q^3 = \left(\frac{1}{6}\right) \left(\frac{5}{6}\right)^3 = \frac{125}{1296}$$

The probability of 0 successes and 4 failures is

$$q \times q \times q \times q = q^4 = \left(\frac{5}{6}\right)^4 = \frac{625}{1296}$$

So the probability of 4 successes in a row is

$$\frac{1}{1296}$$

The probability of 3 successes and 1 failure is

$$4 \times \frac{5}{1296} = \frac{20}{1296}$$

(because there are 4 ways it can happen).

The probability of 2 successes and 2 failures is

$$6 \times \frac{25}{1296} = \frac{150}{1296}$$

(because there are 6 ways it can happen).

The probability of 1 success and 3 failures is

$$4 \times \frac{125}{1296} = \frac{500}{1296}$$

The probability of 0 successes and 4 failures is

$$1 \times \frac{625}{1296} = \frac{625}{1296}$$

Now look, though, as we remind ourselves of a little algebra. Using your knowledge of the binomial expansion, expand $(p+q)^4$

$$(p+q)^4 = p^4 + 4p^3q + 6p^2q^2 + 4pq^3 + q^4$$

This makes a very easy way to solve probability problems based on repeated trials. As we have already seen, a convenient way to obtain the coefficients of the binomial expansion is to note that each coefficient of the expansion can be obtained from the previous term as follows: Multiply the coefficient of the previous term by the exponent of q and divide the result by one more than the exponent of p. Thus, for example, in the expansion

$$(p+q)^8 = q^8 + 8q^7p + 28q^6p^2 + 56q^5p^3$$
$$+ 70q^4p^4 + 56q^3p^5 + 28q^2p^6 + 8qp^7 + p^8$$

we obtain the coefficient of q^6p^2 from the term $8q^7p$ as $(8)(7)/2 = 28$, or the coefficient of q^5p^3 as $(28)(6)/3 = 56$, etc.

The examples that follow are there for those who are interested in strengthening their confidence with probability theory and its ideas. I find that the practice helps.

Study exercises 2

Don't say that I haven't given you enough practice!

Express all the answers representing probabilities as fractions in lowest terms.

1　A card is drawn at random from a deck of 52 playing cards. What is the probability that it is an ace or a face card?

2　If a dice is rolled twice, what is the probability that the first roll yields a 5 or a 6, and the second anything but a 3?

3　In a single throw of two dice, what is the probability that neither a double nor a 9 will appear?

4　In a bag there are 6 white and 5 black balls. If they are drawn out one by one without replacement, what is the chance that the first will be white, the second black, and so on alternately?

5　One man draws three cards from a well-shuffled deck without replacement, and at the same time another tosses a coin. What is the probability of obtaining three cards of the same suit and a head?

6　A man owns a house in town and a cabin in the mountains. In any one year the probability of the house being burgled is 0.01, and the probability of the cabin being burgled is 0.05. For any one year what is the probability that:
   (a) both will be burgled
   (b) one or the other (but not both) will be burgled
   (c) neither will be burgled?

7　The probability that a certain door is locked is $\frac{1}{2}$. The key to the door is one of 12 keys in a cabinet. If a person selects two keys at random from the cabinet and takes them to the door with him, what is the probability that he can open the door without returning for another key?

8　A pair of dice is tossed twice. What is the probability that either a 7 or a 12 appears on the first throw, and that neither a double nor an 8 appears on the second throw.

9　If 3 dice are thrown, find the probability that:
   (a) all 3 will show fours
   (b) all 3 will be alike
   (c) 2 will show fours and the third something else
   (d) only 2 will be alike
   (e) all 3 will be different.

10 How many 4-digit numbers can be formed from the digits 1, 3, 5, 7, 8 and 9, if none of these appears more than once in each number?

11 A girl has invited 5 friends to a dinner party. After locating herself at the table, how many different seating arrangements are possible?

12 From 7 men and 4 women, how many committees can be selected consisting of:
(a) 3 men and 2 women
(b) 5 people of which at least 3 are men?

13 A company has 7 men qualified to operate a machine which requires 3 operators for each shift.
(a) How many shifts are possible?
(b) In how many of these shifts will any one man appear?

14 In how many seating arrangements can 8 men be placed around a table if there are 3 who insist on sitting together.

15 A committee of 10 is to be selected from 6 lawyers, 8 engineers and 5 doctors. If the committe is to consist of 4 lawyers, 3 engineers and 3 doctors, how many such committees are possible?

16 Seven dice are rolled. Calling a 5 or a 6 a success, find the probability of getting:
(a) exactly 4 successes
(b) at most 4 successes.

Chapter 3

Using the normal curve

Parametric statistical analysis

As mentioned earlier, items such as the mean or the standard deviation are known as *parameters*. Hence, any statistical analysis which relies on a connection between such parameters and the probability of events occurring, is called *parametric statistics*. For various reasons, parametric statistical analysis is only approporiate when we have quite large samples and a very large population – and even then, we cannot always use parametric approaches.

One activity of great importance in the analysis of medical data is the attempt to ascertain what the probability of an event occurring is on the basis of sampling. If your research project calls for such an approach, you want to be clear in your own mind whether you are assuming that the distribution of the event in question is *normal* or *binomial*. It might be neither of these, in which case this account will be of less use to you, but happily, most large distributions in medical work come down to one or the other. It is therefore important to know what we mean by a normal distribution and by a binomial distribution. In this chapter we deal with normal distributions.

Normal distribution

A continuous distribution is defined as *normal* if it satisfies a number of mathematical criteria. One of the most important of these is that the area under the curve – that between it and the x-axis – is equal to 1. To be absolutely accurate, it approaches as near as we want to 1, but cannot exceed 1. The reason for this coy language is that the curve never actually touches the x-axis in any finite distance (*see* Figure 3.1). As the curve stretches out to the right and the left, it never actually touches the x-axis except at infinity. The mathematics behind all of this is incredibly beautiful, but well beyond the needs of the readers of this book. But the fact that the total area under the curve gets as close to 1 as it can, and never exceeds it, renders it ideal for describing probabilities because, as you know, the total of any probability space adds up to 1.

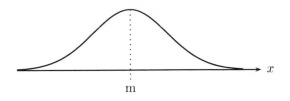

Figure 3.1 The normal curve.

Another important mathematical property of the normal curve is that the area under the curve, between the mean and σ (1 standard deviation to the right) is 0.34. Likewise, the area under the curve between the mean and $-\sigma$ (1 standard deviation to the left) is also 0.34. The normal curve is bilaterally symmetrical about the mean. Thus, we can say that the area trapped under the normal curve between $-\sigma$ and σ is 0.68. All of this becomes easier to appreciate if you examine Figure 3.2. Now you can see that 13% of the area under the normal curve is trapped between σ and 2σ, and another 13% between $-\sigma$ and -2σ. That means that the total area trapped under the curve between the mean and 2σ is 47%, while the area trapped under the curve between the mean and -2σ is also 47%. That is, the total area trapped under the curve between -2σ and 2σ is 94%. Another way of expressing this is

$$m \pm 2\sigma = 0.94$$

Between 2σ and 3σ only 2.5% of the area is trapped. The same is true between -2σ and -3σ. If you add these figures up, you will see that 99% of the area under the normal curve and above the x-axis is trapped between -3σ and 3σ. Now here is where the link with probability theory comes in. Since probability spaces add up to 1, then, if a distribution of health data is

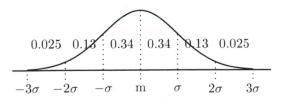

Figure 3.2 Areas trapped under various sections of the normal curve.

normally distributed, we can say that there is a probability of 0.99 that any one score in that distribution will fall within 3 standard deviations of the mean!

The gods smile on health workers in this respect because most health measures that we rely on in epidemiology and public health are normally distributed. A very famous distribution which almost all of us have knowingly (or otherwise) contributed to is the distribution of IQ scores. Most of us have sat the standardised Stanford Binet IQ test at some point in school, and thus contributed our bit to the distribution of scores. IQ testing is a rather complex topic, but without going into detail, the mean of the IQ distribution is set at 100 and the standard deviation is 15 IQ points. Out of the general population then, if you have an IQ of 115, only 16% of the population have a higher score than you do. Think about this for a few moments until you are clear about it. For instance, the probability (over the general population) that a person has an IQ between 115 and 130 (between 1 and 2 standard deviations above the mean) is 0.13. Notice that I emphasised over the general population because if you just considered your colleagues in the course you are doing, that would be a highly biased sample because just to qualify to enter the course, your IQ would probably be in excess of 115. IQ is not always an indicator of academic potential, but the correlation is very strong!

When the infinite is finite

Whenever I have taught health workers about the normal curve, I have had questions about the area under it being 1. The questions hinge on the fact that the area under the curve is always increasing because the two ends of the curve never (in any finite distance) touch the x-axis. This means that whenever one arbitrarily stops graphing the normal curve at either end, more area under the curve can be produced simply by extending the curve past this arbitrary point. How, then, can the total area under the curve never exceed 1?

The explanation this author uses is to show students a far easier infinite series whose sum can never exceed 2. Consider the sum of fractions: $1 + \frac{1}{2} + \frac{1}{4} + \frac{1}{8} + \frac{1}{16} + ...$ and call it F.

$$F = 1 + \frac{1}{2} + \frac{1}{4} + \frac{1}{8} + \frac{1}{16} + ...$$

There is no question that it is an infinite series, so any point at which we stop writing fractions and calculate F will only give us an estimate (and a lower estimate) of F, because it would get bigger the more terms we add. You would assume, I suppose, that since you keep adding bits, the sum could never be 'contained'. Let's see. Start adding.

$$F = 1 + \frac{1}{2} + \frac{1}{4} + \dots$$

$$= 1\frac{3}{4} + \dots$$

$$= 1\frac{3}{4} + \frac{1}{8} + \frac{1}{16} + \frac{1}{32} + \dots$$

$$= 1\frac{3}{4} + \frac{7}{32} + \dots$$

Notice that $\frac{7}{32}$ is less than $\frac{1}{4}$. It misses by $\frac{1}{32}$, so that you still don't reach 2 after adding 6 terms. The next 3 terms are

$$\frac{1}{64} + \frac{1}{128} + \frac{1}{256} = \frac{7}{256}$$

but $\frac{7}{256}$ is less than the required $\frac{1}{32}$, which we need to push the previous sum up to 2.

Maybe, F never reaches 2, however far you go, but gets infinitely close to it. In a very real sense, then $F = 2$. This seems most remarkable, but indeed it is true. There do exist infinite sums with finite answers, and such a one is the area under the normal curve. That area was worked out most ingeniously by the German mathematician, Karl Friedrich Gauss (1777–1855). The fact that the area under it is 1 also makes it ideal for probability studies, because probabilities of alternative events must add up to one. For instance, a person can eat too much carbohydrate, or just the right the amount, or too little. Let us suppose that the probability that the person concerned eats too much carbohydrate is $\frac{1}{3}$ and the probability that they eat just the right amount is $\frac{1}{5}$. Then the probability that they eat too little must be

$$1 - \left(\frac{1}{3} + \frac{1}{5} \right)$$

or

$$1 - \frac{8}{15}$$

or

$$\frac{7}{15}$$

Relating σ to probabilities

Now, the standard deviation of a distribution is a measure of dispersion (a very useful one because of this link it shares with areas under the normal curve) and can be used as a linear measurement of scores away from the mean. For instance, we might have a normal distribution with a mean of 20 and a standard deviation of 3.8. What is the probability that a score of 25.7 or more occurs in that distribution? Note that we have specified that it is a normal distribution. If we cannot safely assume that, then we cannot use any of this attractively useful information!

Well, we are talking about a total deviation from the mean of

$$25.7 - 20 = 5.7$$

How many standard deviations is this? One standard deviation is 3.8 in this distribution, so $\frac{5.7}{3.8} = 1.5$ standard deviations. The probability that it is within one standard deviation of the mean is about 0.68. But that runs from $m - \sigma$ up to $m + \sigma$. Let us only consider m up to $m + \sigma$. That is a probability of about 0.34, so the probability that it lies beyond (further to the right of) $m + \sigma$ is 0.16. I am sure that you will agree that the probability of the score lying to the right of m is 0.5.

Now, the probability that it lies between m and $m + 2\sigma$ is about $\frac{0.95}{2}$ or 0.475. Hence the probability that it lies beyond that is 0.025. So the probability that it is halfway between must be greater than 0.025 and less than 0.16.

Thank heaven, we can do better than that, though. Take a look at the Z-table in Appendix A. Z is the number of standard deviations that a score, x, is away from the mean. Thus

$$Z = \frac{x - m}{\sigma}$$

The values: $m \pm \sigma$, $m \pm 2\sigma$ and $m \pm 3\sigma$ only give us rough methods of estimating relevant probabilities with normal distributions. The Z-table allows us to do it exactly. In the table, under the column A, the proportion of the total area under the curve between the mean and a particular score is given. The figures in A are expressed as proportions of 1, since 1 is the total area. Thus, these convert to probabilities, of course. The Z-tables allow all sorts of interesting applications – provided we can assume that the distributions involved are normal.

Example

In the original example given, our score was 25.7 and σ was 3.8. The mean was 20.

$$Z = \frac{25.7 - 20}{3.8} = 1.5$$

The Z-table shows the areas under the curve associated with each Z-value. The meaning is made clear by the little diagram at the top of the table. Looking up a Z-score of 1.5, we see that it corresponds with a total area of 0.9332. The total area under the curve is 1.0000, so we subtract 0.9332 from 1.0000, which gives us 0.668. Now, how does this compare with our estimates of a value between 0.025 and 0.16 to the right of the mean? Remember, the Z-Table covers the whole area under the normal curve, not just the bit to the right of the mean, so to the figures 0.025 and 0.16 we must add 0.5, making our range of estimate: 0.525 and 0.66. So, we were right, but it is much more useful having an exact figure!

Example

Suppose that daily fluid intake follows a normal distribution in adult females, with a mean of 2500 cc and a standard deviation of 30.2 cc:

(a) What percentage of these women would you expect to ingest at least 2560cc?
(b) What range of values would you expect to include the middle 60% of fluid intakes?

Solution

Always start by sketching a normal distribution and by marking in the relevant values and unknowns, as in Figure 3.3.

$$Z = \frac{2560 - 2500}{30.2} = \frac{60}{30.2} = 1.99$$

The A associated with a Z of 1.99 is 0.4767. Hence the probability of a fluid intake of between 2500 cc and 2560 cc is 0.4767. That means, to have a fluid intake of at least 2560 cc must be $0.5 - 0.4767 = 0.0233$. That gives us what we need to answer part (a). The actual answer is

$$0.0233 \times 100 = 2.33\%$$

The middle 60% range of values has to include the mean, with 30% on either

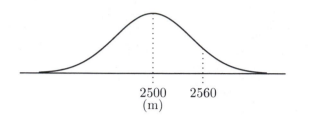

Figure 3.3 For (a) we need the upper tail of the distribution, that to the right of 2560.

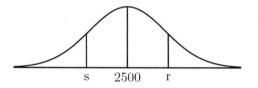

Figure 3.4 The area under the curve between s and 2500 must be 30% and the area under the curve between 2500 and r must be 30%.

side of it. Suppose the upper bound is r and the lower bound is s. Then we are thinking in terms of Figure 3.4. Let us calculate r

$$\frac{r - 2500}{30.2} = 0.84$$

We found that Z-score from checking down until we found an A as close to 30% as we could get, namely, 29.96%. Now, solve the equation for r

$$r - 2500 = 30.2 \times 0.84$$

$$r - 2500 = 25.37$$

$$r = 2525.37$$

Then s must be $2500 - 25.37 = 2474.63$. So 60% of the fluid intakes, the middle 60%, are included in the range 2474.63–2525.37.

Example

In a normal distribution with a mean of 36 and a standard deviation of 5, below what score would 25% of the distribution fall?

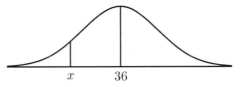

Figure 3.5 The mean 36 and the unknown X shown on the normal curve.

Solution

Here we have a different situation as illustated in Figure 3.5. Let X be the value we want. X must be less than 36 because below 36 lies 50% of the distribution. X has to be the value below which only 25% of the distribution falls. We can, of course, turn the Z-score formula around to keep the values positive

$$Z = \frac{36 - X}{5}$$

But the z-score associated with 0.25 is 0.67, therefore

$$\frac{36 - X}{5} = 0.67$$

$$36 - X = 3.35$$

$$X = 36 - 3.35$$

$$X = 32.65$$

Thus, below a score of 32.65 lies 25% of the distribution.

Chapter 4

An approximation to the normal curve

The binomial distribution

Another distribution commonly used in medical work is the *binomial*. This is particularly applicable to situations in which we know, or strongly suspect, that the probability of a particular event occurring is p and hence that the probability of it not occurring is $q = p - 1$. The binomial distribution is also useful because it is easily adapted so as to be used as 'normal' data, thus allowing access to the various tests already discussed. The problem with the binomial distribution is that it is difficult for non-mathematicians to understand it and to feel at home with it.

Throwing dice

In an attempt to overcome this problem, we shall start with a very routine problem, the rolling of a pair of dice. Each dice has 6 faces – of value (in dots) 1, 2, 3, 4, 5 and 6 respectively. For the sake of argument, let us assume that one dice is red and the other is green: this will become important later in the explanations. Now, what is the probability of both dice scoring 4 when they are rolled simultaneously? The probability of the red one producing 4 is $\frac{1}{6}$, because it could just as easily display any one of its 6 faces. Likewise, the probability of the green one scoring 4 is also $\frac{1}{6}$. Now, what is the probability of both events occurring simultaneously?

All right, we are imagining both dice being thrown together. But before we can even consider the green one, the red one has to score 4. That already excludes $\frac{5}{6}$ of the total probabilities, leaving us only $\frac{1}{6}$ as our total probability out of which to then work out the green ones's chances!

But the green one only has a probability of $\frac{1}{6}$ itself of scoring 4. So that is really $\frac{1}{6}$ of the available probabilities, which is $\frac{1}{6}$ of $\frac{1}{6}$. In other words, the probability that both will score 4 simultaneously is

$$\frac{1}{6} \times \frac{1}{6} = \frac{1}{36}$$

That would be the same with any two independent events. What the green dice does and what the red dice does are independent of each other. Moreover, the 6 events of which each dice is capable are all mutually exclusive, i.e. if a dice rolls 5 that excludes scores of 1, 2, 3, 4 and 6 on that dice.

In a roll of two dice, the possible scores are 2, 3, 4, 5, 6, 7, 8, 9, 10, 11 and 12. Does anyone doubt that? How could you get a score of 1 in rolling 2 dice? Is a score of 13 possible?

Let us now work out the probabilities of each score, the results are shown in the following table.

Score	Dice score Red	Dice score Green	Probability of each pairing	Total probability
2	1	1	$\frac{1}{36}$	$\frac{1}{36}$
3	2	1	$\frac{1}{36}$	$\frac{2}{36}$
	1	2	$\frac{1}{36}$	
4	3	1	$\frac{1}{36}$	$\frac{3}{36}$
	2	2	$\frac{1}{36}$	
	1	3	$\frac{1}{36}$	
5	4	1	$\frac{1}{36}$	$\frac{4}{36}$
	3	2	$\frac{1}{36}$	
	2	3	$\frac{1}{36}$	
	1	4	$\frac{1}{36}$	
6	5	1	$\frac{1}{36}$	$\frac{5}{36}$
	4	2	$\frac{1}{36}$	
	3	3	$\frac{1}{36}$	
	2	4	$\frac{1}{36}$	
	1	5	$\frac{1}{36}$	
7	6	1	$\frac{1}{36}$	$\frac{6}{36}$
	5	2	$\frac{1}{36}$	
	4	3	$\frac{1}{36}$	
	3	4	$\frac{1}{36}$	
	2	5	$\frac{1}{36}$	
	1	6	$\frac{1}{36}$	

Score	Dice score		Probability of each pairing	Total probability
	Red	Green		
8	6	2	$\frac{1}{36}$	$\frac{5}{36}$
	5	3	$\frac{1}{36}$	
	4	4	$\frac{1}{36}$	
	3	5	$\frac{1}{36}$	
	2	6	$\frac{1}{36}$	
9	6	3	$\frac{1}{36}$	$\frac{4}{36}$
	5	4	$\frac{1}{36}$	
	4	5	$\frac{1}{36}$	
	3	6	$\frac{1}{36}$	
10	6	4	$\frac{1}{36}$	$\frac{3}{36}$
	5	5	$\frac{1}{36}$	
	4	6	$\frac{1}{36}$	
11	6	5	$\frac{1}{36}$	$\frac{2}{36}$
	5	6	$\frac{1}{36}$	
12	6	6	$\frac{1}{36}$	$\frac{1}{36}$

Approximating the normal curve

If we draw up a bar graph of this data, a rather interesting similarity with something else you have studied becomes apparent (*see* Figure 4.1). If the data were continuous and we were thus permitted to sketch a curve through the points, we would have a symmetrical curve roughly similar to a normal curve. Likewise, we can use p and q (the probabilities of the event in question occurring or not occurring, respectively), along with n (the number of trials or situations in which the event might or might not occur), to work out the parameters that we use in analysing the normal distribution.

For instance, if you roll one dice 100 times, how many times would you get a 5? One does not have to be all that perceptive (although a rather hairy mathematical proof is required to really establish it) to guess that you would get a 5 about $(100 \times \frac{1}{6})$ times.

In other words, that would represent our 'mean', around which we could 'test' other values. For instance, if on 100 throws, you only get a 5 twice, you should be a bit suspicious! You are comparing 2 with the expected 16.6.

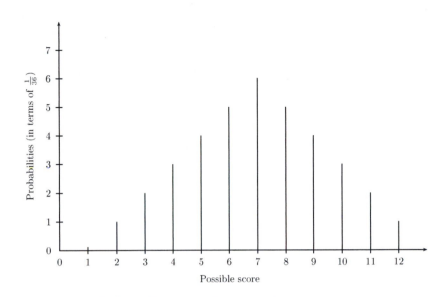

Figure 4.1 Bar graph of all possible scores from two dice.

Again, using some rather high-flown mathematics, we can show that in a binomial distribution, the standard deviation equals

$$\sqrt{n \times p \times q}$$

So the standard deviation of numbers of scores of 5 in 100 rolls of a dice is

$$\sqrt{100 \times \frac{1}{6} \times \frac{5}{6}} = \sqrt{\frac{500}{36}} = 3.73$$

For the purpose of this calculation, we shall assume that everything we are doing is 'legal'!

$$Z = \frac{16.6 - 2}{3.73} - 3.91$$

That is, a score of two 5s in 100 rolls of a dice is going to occur by statistical chance alone in much less than 1 time out of 100. We would reject H_0* and

---

* The reader may not understand that blithe reference to H_0. H_0 means the hypothesis that there is nothing fishy about the dice. It is explained more fully later on.

assume that we were not dealing with an ordinary dice. It has probably been 'weighted' with dishonest intent in mind.

Using the binomial distribution algebraically

Because $p + q = 1$ and because 1 raised to any power is still 1, we can consider another interesting approach to the binomial distribution. Suppose that a couple are advised that there is a probability of 0.25 that if they have a child it will have a hare-lip/cleft palette. Nowadays, this does not have the same dreadful implications that it did in earlier times, and a series of surgical techniques have been elaborated which, in most cases, can allow such a baby to grow to enjoy normal activities and life-style. However, it is a consideration, and a couple given information like that would not enter lightly into a pregnancy without much thought. Remember that we are talking about independent events. Each successive baby is genetically independent of previous babies from the same couple. If the woman had produced a string of 6 normal babies, the chance of the 7th being hare-lip/cleft palette would still be 0.25.

If $p = \frac{1}{4}$ (the probability of hare-lip/cleft palette to that couple), then $q = \frac{3}{4}$ (the probability of a baby without hare-lip/cleft palette). What if the mother had 5 babies? What is the probability of those consisting of 3 hare-lip/cleft palette (let's call those ones H) and 2 without it (call them M)?

$$P(3H, 2M) = ?$$

Don't forget, they can come in any order. It doesn't have to be $HHHMMM$. We could have $HHMHM$, $HMHHM$, $MHHHM$, etc. If we expand the binomial $(p + q)^5$, we can get the answer

$$(p + q)^5 = p^5 + 5p^4q^1 + 10p^3q^2 + 10p^2q^3 + 5pq^4 + q^5$$

The situation we are looking for is p^3q^2, of which there are 10, so the probability we want is given by

$$P(3H, 2M) = 10p^3q^2 = 10\left(\frac{1}{4}\right)^3\left(\frac{3}{4}\right)^2 = 10 \times \frac{1}{64} \times \frac{9}{16} = 0.08789$$

Now, even without the binomial expansion, we could have worked it out, but rather laboriously, as follows

$$P(HHHMM) = \frac{1}{4} \times \frac{1}{4} \times \frac{1}{4} \times \frac{3}{4} \times \frac{3}{4}$$

It doesn't matter how you rearrange the order of the $3H$'s and $2M$'s in the product, the answer will still be

$$\frac{9}{1024}$$

which represents the probability for any given arrangement. All we have to do now is to find some systematic way of listing every arrangement, shown in the table

HHHMM
MHHHM
MMHHH
HMMHH
HHMMH
HHMHM
MHHMH
HMHHM
MHMHH
HMHMH

See! There are 10 ways of doing it, with a probability of

$$\frac{9}{1024}$$

for each possibility. The possibilities, of course, are mutually exclusive, so the probability that in one way or another she will produce 3 hare-lip/cleft palette babies and 2 without it, is

$$10 \times \frac{9}{1024} = \frac{90}{1024} = 0.08789$$

But I think you will agree that it was a lot easier using the binomial expansion. In any case, you cannot always list them in that way. Suppose you had to work out the probability, say, of getting 3 out of 9

$$(p+q)^9 = p^9 + 9p^8q^1 + 36p^7q^2 + 84p^6q^3 + 121p^5q^4$$

$$+ 121p^4q^5 + 84p^3q^6 + 36p^2q^7 + 9p^1q^8 + q^9$$

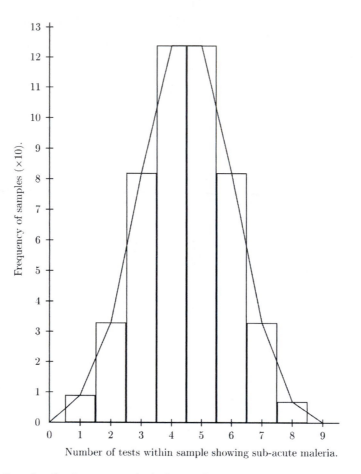

Figure 4.2 Levels of sub-acute malaria in 512 batches of 9 blood samples.

Could you imagine trying to find, by some systematic process, all 84 arrangements of 6 p's and 3 q's!

Example

Among an isolated group of people in the New Guinea Highlands there was reason to believe that blood samples would show sub-acute malaria in 50%. Nine people were tested. What is the probability (using the binomial/normalised approximation) of finding that anywhere from 3 to 6 of the people inclusive were sub-acute malarial? Guidance in the solution of this sort of problem is indicated by a histogram compiled by previous health workers based on testing blood samples in batches of nine. The histogram in Figure 4.2 gives the results for 512 batches.

Solution

To 'normalise' such a situation, we imagine the histogram to have been smoothed over and made continuous. Thus, to consider the interval 3–6, we have to look at the probability of getting 2.5 up to 6.5 sub-acute cases. Then, to obtain the desired probability, we divide this area by 512. Our normal approximations for the relevant parameters are

$$m = np = 9 \times \frac{1}{2} = 4.5$$

and

$$\sigma = \sqrt{9 \times \frac{1}{2} \times \frac{1}{2}} = 1.5$$

For $x = 2.5$

$$Z = \frac{2.5 - 4.5}{1.5} = -1.33$$

For $x = 6.5$

$$Z = \frac{6.5 - 4.5}{1.5} = 1.33$$

The negative part is symmetric with the positive part, so we look up the area from $Z = 0$ to $Z = 1.33$ and double it. The desired probability, then, is given by

$$P = 0.4082 \times 2 = 0.8164$$

Now, how accurate is this normalisation? We can work out the problem entirely in binomial terms and compare the results.

$$\text{Probability of 3 sub-acute cases} = \frac{84}{512}$$

$$\text{Probability of 4 sub-acute cases} = \frac{126}{512}$$

$$\text{Probability of 5 sub-acute cases} = \frac{126}{512}$$

$$\text{Probability of 6 sub-acute cases} = \frac{84}{512}$$

The probability of getting 3–6 sub-acute cases, then, is $\frac{420}{512}$ or 0.8203. As you can see, the discrepancy is not great. Would you expect the discrepancy to increase or decrease as n increased?

Testing statistical hypotheses

Suppose that we have administered an antimalarial prophylactic to our Papua New Guinea Highlanders, and we want to see if it has reduced the incidence of sub-acute malaria. This sort of situation will be discussed in greater detail in the following chapter, when we formally consider null hypotheses. However, for now, we know that we expect 50% of the sample to show sub-acute malaria, and we will be pessimistic and operate under the assumption that our prophylactic has had no effect. That is, when we examine blood smears from the samples who have had the antimalarial prophylactic, we will expect half of them to show sub-acute malaria!

We examine 100 smears, of which only 40 are positive. Can we conclude that the prophylactic has reduced the incidence of sub-acute malaria?

Using the normal curve approximation to the binomial distribution, we get

$$n = 100$$

so

$$m = np = 100 \times \frac{1}{2} = 50$$

and

$$\sigma = \sqrt{100 \times \frac{1}{2} \times \frac{1}{2}} = 5$$

Since we are normalising, hence treating our discrete data as continuous, we test the probability of getting 60 smears sub-acute-free by testing for 59.5 on the Z-scores

$$Z = \frac{59.5 - 50}{5} = 1.90$$

Our probability of getting 60 or more (hence our use of 59.5 rather than 60.5) is thus

$$0.5 - 04713 = 0.0287$$

Therefore, if our prophylactic has had no effect on the incidence of sub-acute malaria, there are still close to 3 chances in 100 of getting samples of size 100 with as many as 60 or more smears clear of sub-acute symptoms.

How are we to interpret such a finding? We are free to interpret it in any way we like. Basically, we could say one of the two things.

1 The prophylactic has had no effect, but just by the pure statistics of the thing we got 60 smears free of sub-acute symptoms. This is only going to happen around 3 times out of 100, but that is a high enough probability for us not to be unduly surprised when it happens.

2 Three out of 100 (2.8 out of 100 actually) is so small that we can safely conclude that its occurrence in our sample indicates that the sample did not come from a population in which half the smears were positive, but from a population with a lower incidence than that. In other words, we can assume that the prophylactic does make a difference.

Which is right? We cannot be sure, but what we do in statistics – and it is particularly important in medical work – is to agree ahead of time on a 'significance level'. If we had said, 'Let us assume that if we get an event in our sample that has only a 5% chance of occurring purely by chance, we will accept that as evidence that something has occurred in our sample to change its characteristics with respect to the attribute concerned', then that would be what we call a significance level of 5%. Had we agreed to a 5% (0.05) significance level before administering the anti-malarial prophylactic, we would have (on the results contained) concluded that the prophylactic was working.

However, it is usual in testing pharmaceuticals to have a lower significance level. 1% (0.01) is the usual. If we had been using that as our level of significance, our prophylactic would have been rejected and we would have had to send the researchers back to their drawing boards!

So the choice of 'level of significance' is arbitrary, even if largely standardised. If we choose a level of significance (we call it α) too high, then we will accept many samples as having reflected a difference when, in fact, they did not – the noted deviance having been due only to random chance. But if we choose α too small, we will end up rejecting treatments as being useless when, in fact, they were effective. To err in the first instance (i.e. accepting a deviance as being due to something we did to the sample, when it was really only due to chance) is called a 'Type 1 error'. To err the other way (i.e. assuming that the deviance obtained is due only to statistical chance and not as a result of our treatment of the sample) is called a 'Type 2 error'.

In medical matters it is clearly more important to reduce Type 1 errors. We do this by setting α at lower values. But do you see that, if you reduce the risk of Type 1 error, you automatically increase the risk of Type 2 error? This is all of such crucial importance that it is dealt with again in the next chapter.

The relationship between binomial and normal distributions

We have seen from the problems discussed in the last few pages, that under certain circumstances we can use the Z-tables of the normal distribution to approximate probability determinations arising in binomial distributions. But we have cunningly refrained from saying what those 'certain circumstances' are. In this section we shall try to unravel that problem.

Suppose you have a probability, p, of 0.01 that an event will occur, say, that a blood smear will contain a trypanosome parasite. Suppose 6 samples are taken. What is the probability that 4 or more of the samples will contain trypanosome parasites?

Clearly this is a binomial phenomenon, so we start with the expansion

$$(p+q)^6 = P^6 + 6p^5q + 15p^4q^2 + 20p^3q^3 + 15p^2q^4 + 6pq^5 + q^6$$

The probability of 4 or more containing trypanosomes is thus given by

$$p^6 + 6p^5q + 15p^4q^2 = (0.01)^6 + 6(0.01)^5(0.99) + 15(0.01)^4(0.99)^2$$

$$= 10^{-12} + 5.94 \times 10^{-10} + 14.7015 \times 10^{-8}$$

$$= 10^{-12} + 0.000000000594 + 0.000000147015$$

$$= 0.000000147610$$

OK, now let's see how it works out using the normal approximation of the binomial distribution

$$m = np = 6 \times 0.01 = 0.06$$

$$sd = \sqrt{npq} = \sqrt{6 \times 0.01 \times 0.99} = \sqrt{0.0594} = 0.24$$

That gives a very skewed distribution – as shown in Figure 4.3.

$$Z = \frac{3.5 - 0.06}{0.24} = \frac{3.44}{0.24} = 14$$

Our own Z-table only goes up to 3 and a bit standard deviations past the mean. If one checks on an extended Z-table though, the probability

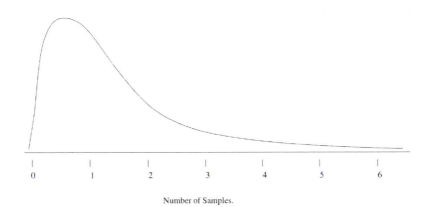

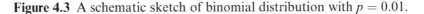

0	1	2	3	4	5	6

Number of Samples.

Figure 4.3 A schematic sketch of binomial distribution with $p = 0.01$.

associated with 14 standard deviations away from the mean is 10^{-5}, which is about 100 times higher than the exact probability on the binomial expansion. What this means is that the normal approximation to the binomial distribution is only appropriate if:

(a) p is reasonably close to $\frac{1}{2}$
(b) n is greater than 50.

The question must now arise: how can we handle binomial-type data that does not satisfy these criteria? It certainly is not practicable to revert to actual · calculation of the binomial expansion with a large n and a small p. Imagine calculating $(0.001 + 0.999)^{100}$! Fortunately there is a way out – even though it may appear a bit fishy if explained by a Frenchman!

I refer, of course, to the 'Poisson' distribution. 'Poisson' is the French word for fish and the Poisson distribution is dealt with in Chapter 8. Generally most students of epidemiology can leave it out, but it is included for completeness and for the benefit of those who wish to pursue the subtleties of the discourse just that bit further. In every class, I have always had one or two who wish to follow up the argument!

Chapter 5

Testing samples

The whole enterprise of sampling is a major preoccupation in health research, and many difficult mathematical problems bedevil it. In doing clinical research, for example, you might want to ascertain the effect of a particular treatment on males over the age of 50 years who are suffering from arthritis of the shoulder. Possibly, you will have difficulty even finding many shoulder arthritis sufferers who are 50 or over and who are also male. Then, on the other hand, you might have access to more than you can possibly test. If the former situation prevails, your sample will need careful scrutiny to make sure that it is not biased.

For instance, if you can only find, say, 36 males over 50 with shoulder arthritis, it could be that there is some factor keeping such people away. Again, that factor might not, of itself, be a bias factor, but then again it could be. It could be that the clinic is in a rural area and hence not many people attend it anyway. That could not be counted as a 'bias' factor, even though it could lead to a sample so small as to make parametric statistical analysis useless.

On the other hand, suppose there was an auto plant nearby and all the male shoulder arthritis sufferers you saw worked in the same section of that plant, doing the same job. This *would* represent a biased sample and one might not be able to generalise from it to the whole population of shoulder arthritis males over 50 years of age. It is possible that the arthritis in your sample is work-related. If your treatment is successful, it might simply be countering some adverse chemical or other environmental agent encountered in the one particular division in the company. The arthritis might be due in some way to the equipment in the factory, the position workers must assume when using it, etc. In that case, a successful outcome to the use of the new treatment might be its unique effect on a single set of muscles. Even more problematic is the fact that maybe the men concerned are anxious to prove work-risk and therefore may be feigning or exaggerating symptoms.

The above are just a few of the very real problems that can affect sampling. The moral of the story, in research design, is to check carefully the sampling procedure you intend to follow. Discuss it with other people with the sole intention of searching out any unperceived sources of bias.

Random samples

We hear a lot about 'random samples' in statistical reporting. What, precisely, does the term mean? In the first place, a sample that you have designed as a method for securing data can hardly be called 'random', if that adjective is intended to modify 'sample'. What it really means is that the method of selecting the sample is as random as you can make it.

A 'random sample', by definition, refers to a set of measures, each one of which is no more likely to occur in the population from which the sample is drawn than is any other similar measure in the population. By devising a random method of selecting the sample, we try to overcome bias in the actual selection.

Social and medical research is full of famous incidents of bias in the selection process. For instance, if you wish to ascertain the incidence of self-diagnosed migraine headaches among menopausal women, you might find (such good fortune rarely attends real-life research projects!) that the local medical facility has a list of 3288 menopausal women. You only want a sample of 200 so, by random numbers (explained below) you select 200 telephone numbers from a list of telephone numbers of the 3288 women concerned. You then telephone each one and ask the relevant questions. This certainly guarantees nearly a 100% return – with written questionaires, 60% is regarded as a good return – and beats going around knocking on doors. Is anything wrong with it? Just about everything!

In the first place, not every woman would have a telephone. Possession of a telephone says something about the socio-economic status of the person, and hence immediately biases the sample. You have no guarantee that people who do not have telephones have fewer migraines because they are not always being pestered by researchers wanting information; or indeed, that they do not have more migraines because, if they are too poor to have a telephone, they have other more pressing financial worries. One could think of many other possible sources of bias if the sample is based on telephone numbers.

But leaving that aside, just how representative are the 3288 women, from which the sample is to be drawn, of menopausal women generally? Don't forget, those 3288 names are on clinical records, so that has excluded all women who have never been to a clinic! That represents a very serious sampling distortion, because migraine headaches might easily be more closely related to general health than to whether or not a person is menopausal.

That all should serve to emphasise the point already mentioned about scrutinising your sampling procedure carefully.

Assignment by random numbers

Appendix F is a table of random numbers. Such a set of numbers is generated in as random a fashion as can be devised. For instance, if you say to someone:

'Think of any 5 numbers!', you will not get a random set of 5 numbers. Any one person usually puts some 'generator' into action when 'thinking of' numbers, so that even after only a few attempts you can often tell 'how' the person is generating their numbers – even though the person concerned is blithely unconscious of it. The 'mechanism' differs from person to person and is highly individualistic. Someone might be able to consciously suspend such a mechanism for 5 or 10 numbers; but, with a large string of 'thinking of any number' it eventually comes into play.

A set of random numbers eliminates that problem and works as follows. Suppose you want to select a sample from, say, 1000 names. Pick any sequence of 1000 numbers in the random table – any unbroken run of 1000 numbers – and assign one to each of the 1000 names. Then select according to some universal property of the numbers, for example all numbers ending with an odd value, or all numbers ending in 5 or whatever. This will generate a sample entirely without reference to the elements in it.

The procedure is not without problems. For instance, you must – prior to the sampling itself – determine a protocol for replacement selection if one or more of those with the right number ending cannot be selected, for example they might be dead or have left the country. Generally, the protocol is something like: 'Use the nearest unassigned number coming next in the list', or 'reduce the sample size accordingly'.

In medical matters it clearly is more important to reduce Type 1 errors. We do this by setting α at lower values. But do you see that, if you reduce the risk of Type 1 errors, you automatically increase the risk of Type 2 errors? This is all of such crucial importance that it is dealt with again in the next section. Before embarking on that, though, test your understanding on the following problem.

Study exercises 3

In a sperm viability test, 450 samples are placed in rows of five. The number of 'positives' in each row were counted and the results are shown below:

Number of positives	Observed frequencies of rows
0	0
1	1
2	11
3	30
4	38
5	10
	90

If the 'positives' are distributed at random among the rows, we could expect a binomial distribution with $n = 5$. Find an estimate of the following.

1 The average number of positives per row.
2 The probability of a single positive.
3 Using the previous answer, calculate the expected frequencies of rows for each number of positives and compare these with the observed frequencies.
4 Draw the histogram for the expected frequencies, and by means of dotted lines show the histogram for the observed frequencies.

Testing a sample

The purpose in selecting a 'random sample' (or, more correctly, in 'selecting a sample randomly') is usually to test it for something with the expectation that you can generalise your finding to the whole population from which the sample was drawn. This frequently comes down to testing means of samples.

In our previous use of the Z-tables, we tested individual scores to ascertain the probability of their occurring – under the assumption of normality and under the assumption that the score in question was, indeed, from that population and not from a different but overlapping one. Now we are going to do something different.

You have a treatment in mind which you think will change (usually improve!) a particular clinical measurement. Now you can do one of several things. Two approaches are very common and will be described here.

You could randomly select two samples of the right kind of patient. For the moment, let us leave out all the problems of how big the samples should be, whether they should be consciously 'paired', etc. To each individual in both samples you appear to accord the same 'treatment', but one of the samples is really not receiving the 'treatment'. If the 'treatment' is administration of a drug, this is easily accomplished by the use of placebos. In that case, statistical rigour is enhanced if you do a double blind trial. The 'subjects' (the people in the two samples) do not know whether or not they have received a placebo or the real thing. Neither do the people who administer the drug know. The only person who knows is the statistician, who has the list of subject numbers and an indication of those who are only getting placebos. Moreover, even the statistician will not look at the list until the results have all been recorded. This approach involves comparing the means of the two samples, after 'treatment' (or placebo) and will be discussed in greater detail under the sections dealing with testing differences between means and also the t-test. Even if that is precisely the sort of research project you have in mind, resist the temptation to jump ahead right away. You will have a much better insight into what you are doing if you keep reading straight on!

The other appraoch is to randomly select one sample only and to accord it the treatment concerned. Take the mean and see how far it is from the mean of the population. Now, this raises problems that testing individual scores did not. Assume all we need to assume – that the scores in the population are normally distributed, that you know the mean, m, of the scores and the standard deviation, σ, of the scores. But you are not testing a score now. You are testing the *mean of a sample of the scores*. Does this make a difference? It most certainly does!

Suppose you had a population of 50 million and you randomly selected a sample size of 1000 from it. Although the figures would be large, I am sure that you appreciate that it is possible to actually determine how many different samples of 1000 you could get from 50 million. The answer is not 50 000, but much more. There are 50 000 samples of 1000 which have no single element in common, but two different samples are different, even if they only differ in 1 element, or 2, or 3, or 4, and so on. You can see the magnitude of the thing!

Without going into the details of how we can exactly calculate the number of such samples, it is enough to realise that there are indeed a very large number of such samples. Now, suppose we calculate the mean of each possible sample. That in itself creates a distribution. How similar is it to the parent distribution of individual scores? Well, here is the answer.

If the parent population is normal, then the distribution of sample means is also normal. As well, if $\bar{X}$ refers to sample mean, the mean of all the $\bar{X}$'s is equal to 'm', the mean of the population of individuals. Very gratifying! Now for the bad news. The standard deviation of all the $\bar{X}$'s is not the same as the standard deviation of all the X's. That is, it is not σ. If you think about it, you would expect the standard deviation of means of samples to be less than σ, because each $\bar{X}$ is, in itself, a 'contracted' or 'compressed' representative of the X's in that sample. Fortunately, as well, the standard deviation of the sample means is related to the sample standard deviation and, logically enough, to the size of the samples concerned. The exact relationship is

$$sd_{\bar{X}} = \frac{sd_X}{\sqrt{n}}$$

where sd_X is the sample standard deviation, not σ, and where n is the sample size.

Commonly, in statistical parlance, the standard deviation of the sample means, is called 'standard error', indicated by se. Thus, in testing our sample mean, the relevant Z-score would be given by

$$Z = \frac{\bar{X} - m}{se}$$

Analysing a test of sample mean

By how much will $\bar{X}$ have to differ from m before we can definitely conclude that our treatment created change? That is to say, even if you did not treat the sample, it is still very unlikely that its mean, $\bar{X}$, would precisely equal m. So how different does $\bar{X}$ have to be from m before we can be absolutely sure that the difference is due to the treatment and not just to a difference that we would expect in the nature of things anyway? Good question!

The answer is: 'You can *never* be absolutely sure'. You are always open to the possibility of two categories of mistake, no matter how careful you are. You might conclude that the difference is due to the treatment when it is just a random difference. As you know, this is what we call a *Type 1 error*. Likewise, you might assume that the difference between m and $\bar{X}$ is not great enough to warrant belief that the treatment caused that difference, when in fact it did! That is what we call a *Type 2 error*. We shall say more about these types of error later, but let us now look at how we decide on whether or not the treatment was responsible.

The null hypothesis

For safety's sake, we have to be painstakingly careful of promoting new treatments. Not only might they be ineffective; they might be actually harmful. Just remember, both Thalidomide and Opren were clinically tested before being released for use! Therefore, we adopt an essentially pessimistic attitude. We say, in effect: 'Let us assume that the treatment makes no difference'. We call this, naturally enough, the 'null hypothesis' and indicate it by H_0. Now we decide on a probability, always a small one, which we will accept as being our significance level α. Let us say that α is 0.01, meaning that the event only has a probability of 1 in 100 of occuring by chance alone. Having decided on an *alpha*, we then agree that if, on testing the sample mean, we find that there is less than probability α of getting such a difference, we will conclude that H_0 is wrong. In effect, what we will be saying is that the treatment did cause the difference because there is only 1 chance in

100 of such a discrepancy occurring by chance alone. The situation is illustrated in Figure 5.1. In certain situations we are only concerned with the amount of deviation, not considering whether the values are greater or less than m. In that case, the α is divided by 2 and is represented by an area at either end of the normal curve, as illustrated in Figure 5.2. Naturally, we refer to the first of these situations as a 'one-tailed test' and to the second as a 'two-tailed test'. Just as H_0 refers to the 'null hypothesis', so H_a refers to the 'alternative hypothesis'. If a is the level of significance then:

1   In a one-tailed test:
  - if the Z-score from our sample mean is associated with a probability *less* than α, the we reject H_0 and accept H_a at the $\alpha = a$ level of significance
  - if the Z-score from our sample mean is associated with a probability *greater* than α, we accept H_0 and reject H_a at the α level of significance.
2   In a two-tailed test:
  - if the Z-score from our sample mean is associated with a probability less than $\frac{a}{2}$, then we reject H_0 and accept H_a at the α level of significance.
  - if the Z-score from our sample mean is associated with a probability more than $\frac{a}{2}$, then we accept H_0 and reject H_a at the α level of significance.

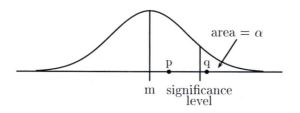

Figure 5.1 A result of p would cause us to accept H_0, while a result of q would cause us to reject H_0.

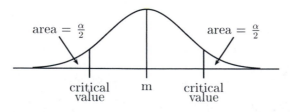

Figure 5.2 Accept H_0 for all values in the interval between the critical values.

Example

From genetics we know that in a certain isolated population, the incidence of thalassaemia (a rare blood disease linked to sickle cell anaemia) is 25%. A group of 228 people whom researchers were not sure as to whether they belonged to the population concerned or not, were tested. 179 of their smears were negative and 49 were positive. Do these figures constitute a significant deviation at the 5% level of significance?

Solution

We would expect, if H_0 were true, that

$$\frac{3}{4} \times 228 = 171$$

people would test negative and 57 would test positive. The figure given in our sample, namely 179 negative, constitutes a deviation of 8 from the expected value. What is the probability of getting a deviation as great (or greater) than 8, that is, 179 or more negative *or* 163 or fewer negative?

Note that the question is concerned with a deviation from the expected. The actual direction of the deviation is not what is important. Thus, we use a two-tailed test.

$$n = 228$$

$$m = \frac{3}{4} \times 228$$

$$= 171$$

$$\sigma = \sqrt{228 \times \frac{3}{4} \times \frac{1}{4}}$$

$$= \sqrt{42.74}$$

$$= 6.54$$

So

$$Z = \frac{178.5 - 171}{6.54} = 1.15$$

on the positive side only.

The probability of that is

$$0.5 - 0.3749 = 0.1251$$

Multiplying it by 2, for both tails gives

$$P = 0.2502$$

Thus, P is well in excess of 0.05 and we can feel quite safe in concluding that the result is not significant. We accept H_0.

Looking at sample means more intuitively

Let us suppose that you really have difficulty making sense of all this sample mean bit. Then carefully consider this problem. Read slowly.

The heights of 1000 Nigerian students were recorded and were normally distributed. The mean height was 68.2 inches with a standard deviation of 2.5 inches. From this group of scores, a sample of 100 was randomly selected. What is the probability that the mean of this sample exceeded 68.9 inches?

If we said: 'What is the probability that a selected student had a height of 68.9 inches or more', the problem would have been easy enough. 68.9 inches is 0.7 inches away from the mean. How big is that interval in standard deviations?

$$\frac{0.7}{2.5} = 0.28$$

The Z-table tells us that the probability of falling between the mean and 0.28 sd's away from it (to the right), the hatched area in Figure 5.3, is 0.1103. But we want to know what the probability of falling beyond that is. We get that by

$$0.5 - 0.1103$$

which is 0.4897. Very nice – but it doesn't answer the original question which was not about an individual student, but about the mean of a sample of 100 students. Well, of course, you can predict the plot from here on, because you already know about that devious $\frac{\sigma}{\sqrt{n}}$ trick, etc., but let's pretend you don't and try to see how far unaided reasoning takes us.

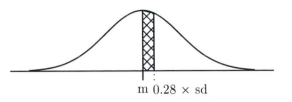

m 0.28 × sd

Figure 5.3 The hatched area corresponds to the probability of falling between the mean and 0.28 sd's above the mean.

Out of 1000, how many different samples of 100 are there? Let's see. How many ways are there of taking 1000 things 100 at a time?

$$1000 \times 999 \times 998 \times \ldots \times 901$$

In other words

$$\frac{1000!}{900!} \div 100! = \frac{1000!}{900!100!}$$

(If you don't recognise that as the number of combinations of 1000 things taken 100 at a time, you need to refer again to Combinations, *see* p. 34.)

$$= \frac{1000 \times 999 \times \ldots \times 901}{100 \times 99 \times 98 \times \ldots \times 1}$$

Never mind calculating it; suffice to say you can get a huge number of different samples of 100 from a population of 1000, certainly more than 1000 samples! Now each of those samples has a mean – no? Moreover and forsooth, those means are normally distributed if the original scores were (*see* Figure 5.4). That's great news! Why is the range of sample means smaller – doesn't extend as far either way – than the range of single scores? Well, think a bit. Suppose that those two dots that you see in Figure 5.5 are the lowest and highest sample means. They couldn't possibly be as far to the left or right as the original scores, because a mean itself implies being in the middle (roughly) of a range. OK? So obviously, the sample means will have less variability than the original population of scores did (*see* Figure 5.6).

Again, as sample size (n) increases, the extreme sample means will draw closer together because 'if you're a little ol' mean in the middle of a big sample, then dang it all, you sho' as hell goin' to be further away from the end score than if you was only in the middle of a small sample!' (as I heard a

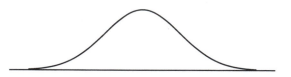

Figure 5.4 Distribution of original scores.

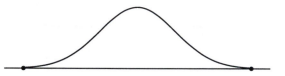

Figure 5.5 Distribution of sample means.

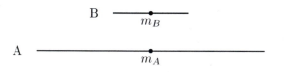

Figure 5.6 The mean of the sample on the left is closer to the ends of its sample than his comrade on the right.

student from Tennessee once say). So, $\frac{\sigma}{\sqrt{n}}$ makes a lot of sense as expressing the standard deviation of sample means, because that $\sqrt{n}$:

- makes the variability less, and
- makes it less and less as n gets bigger and bigger.

But there is yet one more wrinkled orange to throw into the juicer – and this is that all of this only works for sample sizes of 30 or more.

We are safe in treating samples this way as long as our $n \geq 30$. Unfortunately, in epidemiology that is not always possible. The occurrence of samples smaller than 30 requires a different mathematical approach and will be dealt with in Chapter 6. Now we look back at our problem.

The sample is size 100. The ordinary sd is 2.5 inches, so our sample means must have an sd of $\frac{2.5}{\sqrt{100}} = 0.25$. As you know, the short name for 'standard deviation of sample means' is standard error (se). Finding our Z-score in the distribution of sample means, we get

$$Z = \frac{28.9 - 28.2}{0.25} = \frac{0.7}{0.25} = 2.8$$

So the sample mean we are discussing is 2.8 se's from the mean. The area associated with $Z = 2.8$ is 0.4974. So the area (probability) beyond it must be

$$0.5 - 0.4974 = 0.0026$$

Testing a difference of means of large samples

Commonly in medical research we wish to ascertain whether the means of two large samples are significantly different, that is, whether or not they in fact represent two similar populations. H_0, of course, would assert that the difference is not significant and that the two samples are really derived from identical populations. We usually use a two-tailed test in this case, because we are concerned with ascertaining whether the difference (either way) is significant.

Consider two populations, $x_1, x_2, x_3, ..., x_n$ and $y_1, y_2, y_3, ..., y_n$, with means m_x and m_y, and standard deviations σ_x and σ_y, respectively.

The issue becomes a little more hairy (but necessarily so!) if we imagine all the possible samples from the population $x_1, x_2, x_3, ..., x_n$ and all the possible samples from the population $y_1, y_2, y_3, ..., y_n$. In the first population, let us calculate the mean of each of the samples and list them thus: $\bar{x}_1, \bar{x}_2, \bar{x}_3, ...$ In the second population, we do the same: $\bar{y}_1, \bar{y}_2, \bar{y}_3, ...$. For each pair, consider the difference $\bar{x} - \bar{y}$, of sample means. Now, how are these values distributed? It is not hard to show that

$$m_{\bar{x}-\bar{y}} = m_{\bar{x}} - m_{\bar{y}}$$

It is very difficult, however, to prove that

$$\sigma_{\bar{x}-\bar{y}} = \sqrt{se_{\bar{x}}^2 + se_{\bar{y}}^2}$$

and we shall not prove it in this book. It is a useful result in carrying out clinical studies, though. You remember that

$$se_x = \frac{\sigma_x}{\sqrt{n_x}}$$

and

$$se_y = \frac{\sigma_y}{\sqrt{n_y}}$$

For obvious reasons, $\sigma_{\bar{x}-\bar{y}}$ is called the standard error of the differences between sample means or $se_{\bar{x}-\bar{y}}$.

Example

Treatment A is tested on a sample of 50 people which has a mean of 17.0 with a standard deviation of 2.5 with respect to some attribute. Treatment B is tested on a sample of 70 people and, with respect to the same attribute, that sample has a mean of 18.6 with a standard deviation of 3.0. Can we assume that treatment A produces lower means, with respect to the attribute in question, than does treatment B? Note the twist! I have phrased it in such a way as to suggest a one-tailed test.

Solution

In statistics, a sample size of 30 or more is regarded as being large enough to justify the use of normal distribution parameters and Z-scores, providing all other conditions have been met. Chapter 6 considers the situation when sample sizes are less than 30. Now in the particular problem facing us, we do not know the standard deviations of the two populations from which our samples are drawn. But because the sample sizes are relatively large, we shall assume that $\sigma_x = 2.5$ and $\sigma_y = 3.0$.

$$H_0 : m_x - m_y = 0$$

$$\bar{x} = 17$$

$$\bar{y} = 18.6$$

$$sd_x = 2.5, (= \sigma_x)$$

$$sd_y = 3.0, (= \sigma_y)$$

$$n_x = 50$$

$$n_y = 70$$

$$\sigma_{\bar{x}} = \frac{\sigma_x}{\sqrt{n_x}} = \frac{2.5}{\sqrt{50}}$$

$$\sigma_{\bar{y}} = \frac{\sigma_y}{\sqrt{n_y}} = \frac{3.0}{\sqrt{70}}$$

$$\sigma_{\bar{x}-\bar{y}} = \sqrt{\frac{(2.5)^2}{50} + \frac{(3.0)^2}{70}} = 0.5$$

Now we can calculate the Z-score

$$Z = \frac{(\bar{x} - \bar{y}) - (m_x - m_y)}{\sigma_{\bar{x}-\bar{y}}}$$

$$= \frac{(17.0 - 18.6) - 0}{0.50}$$

$$= -3.20$$

Now $|-3.20|$ is greater than 1.96, so the result is significant at the 5% level.

Confidence limits

A closely-related problem to this, and one which likewise has wide application in medical research, is the problem of establishing an interval within which, to a certain degree of confidence, we can say that the mean of a population must fall, purely on the basis of information about samples from that population.

For instance, suppose we took a random sample of 100 from a normally distributed population. The sample had a mean of 40 and a standard deviation of 11. Obviously, we cannot precisely determine the mean of the population because a sample identical to ours could have been taken from any population with a mean close to 40. The very best that we can do is to establish an interval (or limits) within which the population will fall with a stated degree of confidence – almost always expressed as a percentage. Again, it should be obvious that the higher our specified percentage of confidence, the larger will have to be the interval.

In the example cited, we assume that, since the sample is 'large' (over 30) the standard deviation of the population is closely approximated by that of the sample. So

$$se_x = \frac{\sigma}{\sqrt{n}} = \frac{11}{10} = 1.10$$

Now, we are discussing an interval in which the mean lies, so obviously it is a two-tail situation – the interval extending on either side of the true mean.

A Z-value of 1.96 is associated with a significance level of 5%, and hence with a confidence of 95%. Do you understand this connection? In Figure 5.7, if R − S represents the 95% confidence interval in which the mean lies, then

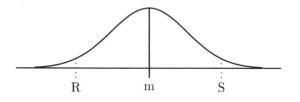

Figure 5.7 The 95% confidence interval.

the area under the curve to the left of R, together with the area under the curve to the right of S, must comprise 5%.

Coming back to our specific problem, we do not know the mean (let us call it 'm') but we want to define it in the interval associated with a *Z*-value of ±1.96. Hence

$$\frac{40 - m}{1.10} = \pm 1.96$$

This creates two equations

$$40 - m = 1.96 \times 1.10 \quad \text{and} \quad 40 - m = -1.96 \times 1.10$$
$$40 - 2.16 = m \quad \text{and} \quad m = 40 + 2.16$$

So our interval is 37.84 to 42.16. This interval has a 95% probability of containing the population mean, assuming that the population itself is normally distributed.

Study exercises 4

1   It has been claimed that 50% of the people have exactly two colds per year. If we decided to reject this claim if among 400 people 216 or more say that they have had two colds per year:
   (a) What is the probability that we have committed a Type 1 error?
   (b) In this investigation, is it possible to commit a Type 2 error? Explain.
2   In a sample of 60 variates the mean is found to be 35 and the standard deviation 4.2. Find the limits within which the population mean is expected to lie with a probability of 98%.

Chapter 6

Testing small samples

Problems with small samples

In dealing with the situation in which we wished to ascertain whether a sample mean was significantly different from the population mean, we – in previous chapters – used a type of Z-score. That is, we divided the difference between m and $\bar{X}$ by the standard error of the mean and used the Z-table (Appendix A) to work out the probabilities. However, all of this assumes not only that the population from which the sample might have been drawn was normally distributed, but that the sample itself was in excess of 30 scores in size.

Obviously, the smaller a sample, the greater is the likelihood that it will be distorted by an extreme value. This makes such ratios as Z increasingly unreliable as the sample sizes decrease. Fortunately, a statistician, William S Gossett, worked out a method of modifying the Z-ratio (he called the modified form 't') so that it can be applied to samples of 30 or fewer. Gosset was the brewmaster for Guiness in Dublin and he needed a test for analysing small samples. However, he felt that he could not publish an academic paper in his position, so he used the pseudonym 'student' in submitting it to mathematical journals. It has therefore since been known, and widely used, as the Student's t-test.

We shall consider four useful medical applications of it.

1　Ascertaining whether the difference between means of paired samples is significant.
2　Ascertaining whether the difference between means of unpaired (independent) samples is significant.
3　Establishing (with some stated degree of confidence) in what interval a population mean lies on the basis of a sample's characteristics. Both this and the next application are considered last and are treated in less detail, because we have already analysed them parametrically.
4　Whether or not a sample mean differs significantly from the population mean.

Two samples

We have already considered the situation in which we compare the mean of a sample with the mean of the population from which it is drawn. What we do in that case, essentially, is to ask: Is $m - \bar{X}$ (or $\bar{X} - m$) so big as to only occur in the normal distribution of the population with a probability of 1 in 100 or less?

Now we shall look at the situation in which you take two samples. It is highly unlikely that the two sample means will be precisely the same, but how large does the difference have to be before we can regard it as significant? In this case we are talking about a distribution made up of differences of sample scores. To analyse it, we clearly have to know what the mean of this new distribution is and what its standard deviation is.

The t-test

There are several ways of approaching this problem and others will be considered in a subsequent chapter, but for now we shall just discuss the t-test method. In order to apply this interesting test, we assume, of course, that the distributions of the two samples are normal and that their standard deviations are equal. We also must have both samples of the same size and with measurements paired. What this means is that each element in your first sample is paired with one, and only one, from the second sample. For instance, this set-up could constitute sets of two measurements on the same subject taken under different conditions, or something similar.

In medical practice, we do not often take children's temperatures orally because of the risk that the thermometer will be chewed. Commonly, the rectum is the 'site of choice' in such cases. We also know that rectal temperature usually differs from oral temperature in the same subject, but is this difference significant? It should be noted that in rural areas of third world countries, the glass mercury thermometer is still routinely used. Ten children were tested as shown in the table below.

Child	Anus	Mouth	Difference (mouth–anus)	(Difference)^2
1	36.2	37.0	0.8	0.64
2	35.7	37.2	1.5	2.25
3	36.0	37.0	1.0	1.00
4	36.4	37.0	0.6	0.36
5	35.8	37.3	1.5	2.25
6	36.2	37.1	0.9	0.81
7	36.1	37.1	1.0	1.00
8	36.5	37.0	0.5	0.25
9	36.5	37.2	0.7	0.49
10	36.4	36.9	0.5	0.25

Notice what we have done with the data obtained. For each pair we calculate the difference (d) and then square each difference. If we then calculate the mean of the differences, we get

$$\frac{\Sigma d}{10} = \frac{9}{10} = 0.9$$

Now we calculate the standard deviation of the d-values. We can do this either by

$$\sqrt{\frac{\Sigma(d_i - \bar{d})^2}{n - 1}}$$

or

$$\sqrt{\frac{\Sigma d^2 - \dfrac{(\Sigma d)^2}{n}}{n - 1}}$$

The second version is more appropriate to the way our data presents, although obviously they are both the same (*see* Chapter 1).

$$\Sigma d^2 = 9.3$$

and

$$(\Sigma d)^2 = (9)^2 = 81$$

So

$$sd = \sqrt{\frac{9.3 - \dfrac{81}{10}}{9}}$$

$$= \sqrt{\frac{9.3 - 8.1}{9}}$$

$$= \sqrt{\frac{1.2}{9}}$$

$$= \sqrt{0.1333}$$

$$= 0.365$$

Actually calculating 't'

All that we have done so far is to calculate the mean and the standard deviation for the peculiar distribution made up of sample mean differences. We will now consider the distribution made up of differences of scores from paired samples. In fact, 't' is given by

$$t = \frac{1/d}{\frac{sd}{\sqrt{n}}}$$

so, in our case

$$t = \frac{0.9}{\frac{0.365}{\sqrt{10}}}$$

$$= \frac{(0.9)\sqrt{10}}{0.365}$$

$$= \frac{(0.9)(3.16)}{0.365}$$

$$= 7.797$$

Now look up the *t*-value table (Appendix B). Notice that there is a column marked 'degrees of freedom'. What does that mean? You will recall that, in accounting for why we divided by $(n - 1)$ instead of just by n in calculating sample standard deviations, the concept of 'degrees of freedom' was addressed. We use $(n - 1)$ because, by calculating the mean, we already 'freeze' one of the values and hence we lose a degree of freedom.

For the same reason, our degrees of freedom are crucial with the t-distribution. We are, after all, restricted to 30 or fewer as a sample size. So, in our case, our degrees of freedom are only 9. As well, we are interested in a one-tail test because we want to know if the oral temperature is significantly higher than the rectal temperature – not if they are (either way) merely significantly different. Therefore, looking along column 9, we see that at the 5% significance level, our *t*-value should be at least 2.2622. Well, ours is 7.797, so we can conclude that at the 5% significance level, our result certainly is significant. It is not necessary to check it at the 1% significance level. Why?

Another application of the t-distribution

The t-test provides a method for ascertaining the relationship between the means of two *independent* samples. The one that we have just dealt with in such detail concerned two *dependent* samples in that each pair represented measures of two different things done to the same person.

In the situation involving two independent samples, we assume also that both samples are distributed normally and that their standard deviations are equal. but the samples do not have to be of the same size.

Here is an example. Suppose you wish to see if there is any significant difference between men's resting systolic pressure and that of women. Stated in that way, would this be a one-tailed or a two-tailed test? We have a sample of 11 men and a sample of 12 women.

Men: 100, 130, 125, 140, 125, 112, 120, 140, 110, 145, 140

Women: 125, 90, 110, 115, 120, 115, 125, 110, 120, 120, 130, 115

Now, these different-sized samples introduce an interesting wrinkle. Let us get them organised first. We will call the size of the smaller sample (men) n_1 and the size of the larger sample (women) n_2. So $n_1 = 11$ and $n_2 = 12$. The value for t that we use is

$$t = \frac{\bar{X}_1 - \bar{X}_2}{\sqrt{sd^2 \left(\frac{1}{n_1} + \frac{1}{n_2} \right)}}$$

But how do we get the sd of both samples combined? This is given by

$$sd = \sqrt{\frac{\Sigma X_1^2 - \dfrac{(\Sigma X_1)^2}{n_1} + \Sigma X_2 - \dfrac{(\Sigma X_2)^2}{n_2}}{n_1 + n_2 - 2}}$$

In fact, you will notice that our degrees of freedom must be $(n_1 + n_2 - 2)$ because we lose one degree of freedom for each sample mean that we calculate. It goes without saying, of course, that $\bar{X}_1$ is the mean of the first sample and $\bar{X}_2$ is the mean of the second sample.

The reader may be somewhat daunted at the prospect of calculating entities such as $(\Sigma X_1)^2$ with such large numbers. However, the relationship between the numbers is not changed if we subtract the lowest score from all the scores. By subtracting 90 from each score, this would give us:

Sample 1: 10, 40, 35, 50, 35, 22, 30, 50, 20, 55, 50

Sample 2: 35, 0, 20, 25, 30, 25, 35, 20, 30, 30, 40, 25

X_1	X_1^2	X_2	X_2^2
10	100	35	1225
40	1600	0	0
35	1225	20	400
50	2500	25	625
35	1225	30	900
22	484	25	625
30	900	35	1225
50	2500	20	400
20	400	30	900
55	3025	30	900
50	2500	40	1600
		25	625
397	16459	315	9425

$$\bar{X}_1 = \frac{397}{11} = 36.09$$

$$\bar{X}_2 = \frac{315}{12} = 26.25$$

So

$$sd^2 = \frac{16459 - \dfrac{397^2}{11} + 9425 - \dfrac{315^2}{12}}{11 + 12 - 2}$$

$$= \frac{16459 - 14328.09 + 9425 - 8268.75}{21}$$

$$= \frac{2130.91 + 1156.25}{21}$$

$$= \frac{3287.16}{21}$$

$$= 156.53$$

Now we can work out the t-value

$$t = \frac{36.09 - 26.25}{\sqrt{156.53 \cdot \left(\frac{1}{11} + \frac{1}{12}\right)}}$$

$$= \frac{9.84}{\sqrt{156.53 \cdot \left(\frac{23}{132}\right)}}$$

$$= \frac{9.84}{\sqrt{27.2742}}$$

$$= \frac{9.84}{5.22}$$

$$= 1.89$$

We are now able to check this at either the 5% or the 1% level of significance, using the t-table as a two-tailed test and with 21 degrees of freedom. At the 5% level of significance, a score in excess of 2.0796 would have to have been obtained in order for the difference between the systolic pressures in our samples of men and women to be significant. Our 't' was only 1.89, which means that the difference was not significant. If it were not significant at the 5% level, then it certainly would not be significant at the 1% level!

In a subsequent chapter, we shall consider some non-parametric tests for similar sorts of situations. Remember that some data that arises in medical research does not conform to a normal curve and thus cannot legitimately be analysed by parametric techniques. If we do not wish to commit ourselves to any assumption as to the normality of data, then we use non-parametric tests.

Establishing an interval for the population mean

This is the issue of confidence (or fiducial) limits which we discussed in the parametric context. An interesting application of its use with small samples is to be found in the summer issue of the *British Medical Journal*, 1979. It is known that Everley's syndrome* generally causes a reduction in blood sodium concentration. Eighteen cases only were described and their mean blood sodium concentration was 115 mmol/l, with a standard deviation of

* A fortunately rare, and congenital blood disease, often causing reduction in concentrations of blood sodium.

12 mmol/l. The question arose: In what range of values might one be 95% certain that the population mean will lie?

Well, our standard error (se) is given by

$$\frac{sd}{\sqrt{n}} = \frac{12}{\sqrt{18}} = 2.83$$

To find the 95% confidence interval for the population mean, then, we need to ascertain a multiple of the standard error. Our degrees of freedom are 17, being 18 − 1, and we use the two-tailed distribution. The *t*-value (from the table in Appendix B) is 2.1098 at the 5% level of significance. Why do we use the 5% level of significance? Simply because we are establishing 95% confidence limits. So, we must multiply our standard error (2.83) by 2.1098 and then establish the interval made by respectively subtracting and adding that value to the mean (115), to get the 95% confidence interval.

$$115 \pm 2.1098 \times 2.83 = 115 \pm 5.97$$

Thus, the population mean lies in the interval 109.03 up to 120.97 with 95% probability. If we wanted to establish a 99% confidence interval, obviously we would use the 1% level of significance in the same way.

Comparing a sample mean with the population mean

We can address this problem by continuing to use the *British Medical Journal* data on Everley's syndrome. Estimates of the plasma calcium concentration yielded a mean of 3.2 mmol/l in our sample of 18. Previous experience from other studies, we are told, states that the mean is usually close to 2.5 mmol/l in healthy people of the same age range. All right – is the mean of the *BMJ* sample exceptionally high? This, of course is a one-tailed test.

$$t = \frac{m - \bar{X}}{se} = \frac{2.5 - 3.2}{0.26} = 2.69$$

Again, using 17 degrees of freedom and a 5% significance level, we get a *t*-value (from the table in Appendix B) of 1.7396. Therefore, at the 5% level, our result certainly *is* significant. At that level, the *t*-value is 1.740, so our result of 2.69 (we take the absolute value, of course) is *not* significant.

Why demand equal standard deviations?

In all the tests comparing pairs of samples that we have explored in this chapter, one of the assumptions has been that their sample standard deviations be equal. Why is this so? For instance, suppose you tried to establish whether or not drinking coffee prior to an examination improved performance. You might find that the mean of sample A (did not have coffee) was the same as the mean of sample B (did have coffee), but that there was a much greater spread of scores in sample B than in A. That is, their sample standard deviations were very different.

This would suggest that, had we compared sample A with sample B by a difference of means test, we would have found no significant difference, and accepted the null hypothesis. On the other hand, suppose one population P is much more widely dispersed than another, S (they are different populations) and we take a sample from each to compare them. But, we don't know that we have picked samples from two different populations. The variability of population P is such that the mean of a sample from it might or might not be close to the mean of the sample from S.

Thus, you can appreciate that the greater the difference in dispersion (and standard deviation is our usual measure for that) between two samples, the less accurately we can come to any conclusion about differences between their means. Hence, the t-tests specify that we assume equal sample standard deviations.

Chapter 7

A taste of epidemiology

What is epidemiology?

The exact tabulation and analysis of patterns of disease spread throughout populations is what is generally involved in epidemiology. In technical terms, the definition is: the study of disease, and of disease attributes, in defined populations. Thus, it deals with both the distribution and the aetiology of disease. Originally, about a century ago, it was concerned solely with such rapidly contagious diseases as typhoid and cholera. Today, epidemiology also embraces the study of non-communicable diseases, as well as contagious diseases.

Malaria kills 20 million people per year and is thus economically important. It is certainly being widely studied in epidemiological terms. Another current object of considerable epidemiological interest is HIV/AIDS.

In short, we can say that epidemiology is the scientific basis for public health and the bedrock of preventive medicine.

Various proportions and rates

We have to have some means of facilitating comparison of the impact of various disease states on populations. With that end in view, note the following words and phrases in particular.

1 *Percent*. This specifies the number out of each 100. Thus, 37% means 37 out of each 100. 37% of 200 would be 74; of 500 would be 185; of 50 would be 18.5, etc.
2 *Prevalence*. This refers to the number of cases at any given time, expressed as a ratio of the number of cases to the number of people in the population of interest at that time.
3 *Incidence*. This indicates the number of *new* cases that occur over a specified time interval. It is usually (but not always) measured as the number of new cases occurring during a period out of the number of people initially at risk of developing the disease.

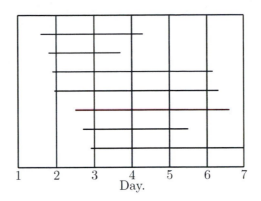

Figure 7.1 Seven cases of a disease reported over time.

Suppose that the number of cases of impetigo occurring in a population of 658 infant school children was 63 over a 12-month period, the incidence (I) would be

$$I = \frac{63}{658} = 0.096$$

If this is taken as a ratio of each 100 children initially at risk, we have

$$I = 0.096 \times 1000 = 96$$

Students often have difficulty in differentiating between incidence and prevalence, but Figure 7.1 should clarify the matter. In Figure 7.1, we assume that each line segment represents a case of the disease in question from onset until it has run its course. On any given day, let us also assume that 1000 people are at risk.

For day 1 the incidence is 4 cases per 1000 persons and for day 2 the incidence is 3 cases per 1000. But, at the end of day 1 the prevalence is 4 per 1000, while at the end of day 2 the prevalence is 7 per 1000. Can you appreciate that two diseases could have identical incidences and yet one of them have a far higher prevalence if its duration is longer?

Incidence measures the rate at which a disease is developing. It can be a useful piece of data in trying to work out the reason for the disease's occurrence. For instance, you can probably think of current examples in which the incidence of a disease is analysed in various sub-populations in order to ascertain why it favours some groups over others.

On the other hand, prevalence measures the actual amount of disease in the population at a given time. We have seen that prevalence is a function of the duration of a disease. It is therefore of great use in planning healthcare facilities for that disease.

We could, but will not, consider various other commonly used ratios in epidemiology, such as the relative risk (RR) and the odds ratio (OR). Instead, let us look at some of the more inferential type phenomena.

Sensitivity, specificity and predictive value

We shall first define these three terms, all of which relate to testing for disease. The *sensitivity* of a test is the proportion of those who have the disease in question and do, in fact, test positive for it on the test used. Beware of the subtlety here. If you get a positive response to a BCG test, it could be because you really do have TB – in which case, the BCG test has worked. But no test is perfect and maybe you don't have TB. In that case, your result is a 'false positive'.

If that can happen, then obviously things can go wrong the other way. You get a negative response to the BCG test, but maybe you really do have TB.

Thus, our definition for sensitivity (as well as for the other two) is based on criteria which the doctor (or other health worker) cannot know. It says, 'The proportion of those who have the disease . . . .'. By that, it does not mean those who tested positive by whatever test was being used, but those who actually have the disease whatever the test says. Bear this in mind when working with these definitions. It's a little like the atheist and the theologian arguing about the existence of God. The actual existence or not of God is independent of them. The theologian, getting nowhere fast in the argument, could well turn round and say, 'He knows you're there even if you don't know He's there!'

Meanwhile, back on the farm . . . .

The *specificity* of a test is defined as the proportion of those without the disease and who, in fact, have tested negative on the relevant test.

And finally, predictive value. The *predictive value* of a test is defined as the proportion of those who, having tested positive, actually do have the disease. Perhaps the table below will clarify things.

Disease status	Tested positive	Tested negative	Total
Absent	980	8820	9800
Present	180	20	200
Total	1160	8840	10 000

From the table we can now calculate our three entities:

$$\text{Sensitivity} \qquad \frac{180}{200} = 0.9$$

$$\text{Specificity} \qquad \frac{8820}{9800} = 0.9$$

$$\text{Predictive value} \ \frac{180}{1160} = 0.155$$

Also $\frac{8820}{8840} = 0.009$. Thus, in a rare disease, high specificity and high sensitivity are not sufficient to ensure that a large proportion of those who tested positively actaully do have the disease. Now that's a turn-up for the books for you.

More informed sectioning of probability spaces

Well, in this brief journey into the realms of epidemiology, we have considered some basic definitions of ratios and some definitions of inferential terms. We shall now attempt to marry all that to what you have already learned (in Chapter 2) about probability. Please take a deep breath and fasten your seat belts – turbulence ahead!

Joint probability

You already know that for any two events, A and B, the probability of one or the other occurring, is given by

$$P(A \ or \ B) = P(A) + P(B) - P(A \ and \ B)$$

I mean, suppose A is: 'You have blonde hair' and B is: 'You play the oboe', then the probability of A *or* B is surely higher then the probability of A *and* B. In a Venn diagram (Figure 7.2) it is easier to see the implications. In Figure 7.2, all the horizontally striped area (all the region in circle A) represents every situation in which the statement: 'You have blonde hair' is a true statement. Likewise, all the vertically striped area (all the region in circle B) represents every situation in which the statement: 'You play the oboe' is a true statement. But A and B overlap. The overlapped region (identifiable as the cross-hatched both horizontally and vertically) must represent the conditions when 'You have blonde hair and you play the oboe'.

Where does 'or' fit in?

Well, look at the numbers 1, 2, 3, and 4 in Figure 8.2. The '1' is not in either circle. It must refer to a situation in which you do not have blonde hair and

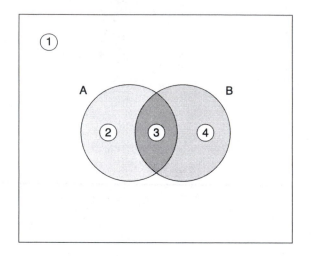

Figure 7.2 Venn diagram of A *or* B.

you also do not play the oboe. The '2' is in A alone and would apply if the
statement: 'You have blonde hair or you play the oboe' was true. Likewise,
'3' would occur in the 'or' case, as would '4'.

If you imagine that each of A and B is a plastic disc overlapped as shown,
the overlapped part would be of double thickness. To get the total region of A
or B, you don't want to include that double thickness. Thus

$$A \ or \ B = A + B - (A \ and \ B \ \text{overlap})$$

In probability terms, each region stands for the probability (taken as a
proportion of the whole area of the rectangle of the Venn diagram) of the
event it represents occurring.

Thought of that way, it is easy to see that

$$P(A \ or \ B) = P(A) + P(B) - P(A \ and \ B)$$

By the simplest exercise of algebraic manipulation, you can see that this also
means that

$$P(A \ and \ B) = P(A) + P(B) - P(A \ or \ B)$$

See if you can also argue that second equation from the original Venn
diagram. Stop now and try it. These two equations, then, represent what we
call 'joint probability'.

Conditional probability

Now look again at Figure 7.2 and see if you can work out, or even conceive of, the probability that B will occur given that A has already occurred. This strange concept, symbolised by the notation

$$P(B|A)$$

is of very great importance in epidemiology and is called 'conditional probability'.

Now let us try to work out what $P(A|B)$ must mean. It would mean, using our Venn diagram: What is the probability that you play the oboe, given that you are blonde? In other words, if you stay in circle A, what proportion of that region is occupied by B? If you understand that, then you are getting somewhere.

The part of A occupied by B is the cross-hatched vertical/horizontal-lined sliver which is the (A and B) region in Figure 7.2. Thus, the probability of B, given that you are to stay in A, must be the ratio

$$\frac{A \ and \ B}{A}$$

Is that clear? If it isn't, don't be discouraged. Just re-read from the 'Conditional probability' section. Therefore

$$P(A|B) = \frac{P(A \ and \ B)}{P(A)}$$

Again, by simple algebra, this can be rearranged as

$$P(A \ and \ B) = P(A) \times P(A|B)$$

We can immediately apply this concept to what we have said about sensitivity and specificity:

$$\text{Sensitivity} = \text{P(test positive/disease present)}$$

$$\text{Specificity} = \text{P(test negative/disease absent)}$$

Dependent and independent events

If two events are independent of one another, what precisely does that mean? It is really difficult to think of two physiological events (in the same person) that are 'independent' because whatever happens to one part of the organism must have some effect on any other event in any other part of the organism, no matter how indirect. In epidemiology, though, we do speak of independent medical events, strictly in mathematical terms.

We can better appreciate how we do this, by using playing cards. That greatly reduces the possibility of messy physiological interconnections.

If you draw an ace from the deck, the fact that it is an ace does not affect its suit, and vice versa. We can certainly say that occurrence of aces (as opposed to non-aces) is an event *independent* of the occurrence of hearts (as opposed to any other suit).

Let A mean 'an ace is drawn' and B mean 'a heart is drawn'. First of all, what would $P(A|B)$ be? We are asked: 'What is the probability of drawing an ace, given that the cards concerned are all hearts?'

Well, there are 13 hearts: 2, 3, 4, 5, 6, 7, 8, 9, 10, J, Q, K, A. Only one of them is an ace, so

$$P(A|B) = \frac{1}{13}$$

But what is $P(A)$? In other words, what is the probability of drawing an ace with no conditions, an ace from the whole pack? There are 4 aces, so

$$P(A) = \frac{4}{52} = \frac{1}{13}$$

Thus, if A and B are independent events, then

$$P(A) = P(A|B)$$

In epidemiology, then, that is how we shall define independent events.

That is not our only test for independence of events, however. Let us imagine that you draw a card and then roll a dice. Dice, like cards, are good because their behaviour is not obscured by physiological inter-relationships.

Obviously, the roll of the dice and the drawing of the card are independent events. OK then. What is the probability of drawing a king and then rolling a 3?

$$P(\text{king}) = \frac{1}{13}$$

$$P(3) = \frac{1}{6}$$

What is P(king and 3)? Well, if you don't draw a king, you don't bother proceeding any further. Thus, there is only $\frac{1}{13}$ of a chance of the probability of the second event being taken into account. Therefore

$$P(\text{king } and \text{ 3}) = \frac{1}{13} \times \frac{1}{6}$$

So, another test for independence of the two events A and B is this: A and B are independent if

$$P(A \text{ and } B) = P(A) \times P(B)$$

Is 'independence' of two events the same as them being 'mutually exclusive'? Many people carelessly think so, but how could that be? Drawing a king cannot prevent the 3 from being rolled, can it?

Application to disease states

Let us consider two diseases, disease A and disease B, in a given population. We will further assume that there is something about these diseases that makes them mutually exclusive – i.e. they cannot occur in the same person. This is not at all fanciful. Sickle cell anaemia and malaria constitute (almost) such a pair. Thus, in our population, disease A does occur and so does disease B, but never together in the same person. Thus

$$P(A \text{ and } B) = 0$$

But P(A) is a positive value and so is P(B). Therefore

$$P(A) \times P(B) \neq 0$$

This shows that two mutually exclusive events are not independent events.

We move onto some real epidemiological data. Among white people, 44% have type A blood (and 56% do not); 14% have type B blood (and 86% do not). But only 3.9% have type AB blood. Are blood types A and B independent traits?

$$P(A) \times P(B) = 0.44 \times 0.14 = 0.06$$

$$P(A \ and \ B) = 0.039$$

Therefore, we can say that they are not independent traits because, if they were P(A and B) would (closely) equal $P(A) \times P(B)$.

Now consider the following problem. A haemophilia-carrying female marries an unaffected male and transmits the disease to half her sons, but to none of her daughters. (Half her daughters will be carriers, though.) What is the probability that she will bear a haemophilic child?

The haemophilic child might be of either sex. So

$$P(\text{affected child}) = P(\text{affected male}) + P(\text{affected female})$$

$$= P(\text{son } and \text{ affected})+$$

$$P(\text{daughter } and \text{ affected})$$

At this point, recall that

$$P(A|B) = \frac{P(A \ and \ B)}{P(A)}$$

and apply it. Our equation should now read

$$P(\text{affected child}) = P(\text{son}) \times P(\text{affected|son})+$$

$$P(\text{daughter}) \times P(\text{affected|daughter})$$

$$= \frac{1}{2} \times \frac{1}{2} + \frac{1}{2} \times 0$$

$$= \frac{1}{4}$$

So the probability that she will have an affected child is $\frac{1}{4}$. Suppose that she considers all of these mathematical implications and decides to have an amniocentesis done to ascertain the sex of the foetus. It turns out that she is carrying a male foetus.

$$P(\text{affected child}|\text{son}) = \frac{P(\text{son } and \text{ affected})}{P(\text{son})}$$

$$= \frac{\frac{1}{4}}{\frac{1}{2}}$$

$$= \frac{1}{2}$$

Apparent anomalies

This branch of statistics is full of all sorts of seeming anomalies that fly in the face of common sense. Just to illustrate the point, let us look at three rather amusing applications of probability theory. Each is presented as a 'discussion item' and should be read and considered as such.

Discussion item 1 – cancer test

- The test is 0.98 accurate.
- If someone has cancer, the test will detect it 98% of the time. If they don't, then the test won't detect cancer 98% of the time.
- Assume that 0.5% (one out of every 200 people) actually has cancer.
- You took the test and got a positive reading. Should you be depressed? Or how depressed should you be!?
- If 10 000 tests are administered there will be 50 cancer sufferers among them and 49 of them will be picked up by the test.
- 9950 will be cancer-free, but 2% of them will test positive. That is, 199 false positives.
- That makes a total of 199 + 49 = 248 positive results. The probability then of having cancer and of having tested positive is

$$\frac{49}{248} = about \ 0.2$$

- Consider condom ads, pap smears, etc.

Discussion item 2 – AIDS and heterosexual encounters

Likelihood of acquiring AIDS heterosexually:

- If partner has AIDS, probability that the other will get it in one episode is $\frac{1}{500}$.

- Therefore the probability of not getting it is $\frac{499}{500}$.
- Therefore the chance of not falling victim in N encounters is $\frac{499}{500}N$.
- $\left(\frac{499}{500}\right)^{364} \approx \frac{1}{2}$.
- Therefore one runs a 50% risk of not getting AIDS if one has intercourse with an AIDS-infected partner every day for a year.

Discussion item 3 – investment advice service

A company advertises an outstanding deal. For 6 weeks running, it will give you a free prediction as to how to invest – free, gratis, no payment. The prediction will say that the index will rise or fall – no pussy-footing.

If they are correct every time, will you pay them 100 pounds to give the investment advice for the next week?

Be careful! If the promoter were a complete charlatan who knew nothing about investments, he could send out the offer to 1 000 000 people. For many of them his prediction will be correct, and they will eagerly check at the end of week 2. Again, he will be right for some. By the end of week 6, he will have been right six times in a row for some people. Those people wouldn't know about his failures, so they would gladly send in their money!

Study exercises 5

1 For a particular population, the lifetime probability of contracting glaucoma is approximately 0.007 and the lifetime probability of contracting diabetes is approximately 0.020. A researcher finds (for the same population) that the probability of contracting both of these diseases in a lifetime is 0.0008. For the next three questions choose one of the following probabilities.

A 0.0400
B 0.0278
C 0.0296
D 0.0262
E 0.1143

(a) What is the lifetime probability of contracting either glaucoma or diabetes?
(b) What is the lifetime probability of contracting glaucoma for a person who has, or will have, diabetes?
(c) What is the lifetime probability of contracting diabetes for a person who has, or will have, glaucoma?

2 On the basis of the information given, which of the following conclusions is most appropriate for the two events: contracting glaucoma and contracting diabetes?

(a) They are independent.
(b) They are not independent.

3 A certain operation has a fatality rate of 30%. If this operation is performed independently on three different patients, what is the probability that all three operations will be fatal?

A 0.09
B 0.90
C 0.009
D 0.027
E 0.27

4 If two-thirds of patients survive their first myocardial infarction and one-third of these survivors is still alive 10 years after the first attack, then among all patients who have a myocardial infarction, what proportion will die within 10 years of the first attack?

A 1/9
B 2/9
C 1/3
D 2/3
E 7/9

5 If 30% of all patients who have a certain disease die during the first year, and 20% of the first-year survivors die before the fifth year, what is the probability that an affected person survives past 5 years?

A 0.50
B 0.10
C 0.56
D 0.06
E 0.14

6 Suppose that 5 men out of 100 and 25 women out of 10 000 are colour-blind. A colour-blind person is chosen at random. What is the probability that the randomly chosen person is male? (Assume males and females to be in equal numbers.)

A 0.05
B 0.25
C 0.75
D 0.95
E 0.99

Chapter 8

From binomial to Poisson

Rates of occurrence

In public health we often need to measure the rate at which an event occurs, such as how often in a series of DNA samples a particular configuration appears or how often in families of a given size a particular ratio of boys to girls among their offspring presents. By way of example, let us ask: In a family of six children, what is the probability that 4 will be boys and 2 girls? (*see* p. 26).

If $p =$ probability of a boy and $q =$ probability of a girl, we are dealing with the binomial expansion

$$(p + q)^6 = p^6 + 6p^5q + 15p^4q^2 + 20p^3q^3 + 15p^2q^4 + 6pq^5 + q^6$$

The particular term we are interested in is the one involving p^4q^2, which is

$$15p^4q^2$$

Under normal circumstances the probability of boys and girls are each $\frac{1}{2}$, so the probability is

$$P \text{ (4 boys and 2 girls)} = 15\left(\frac{1}{2}\right)^4 \left(\frac{1}{2}\right)^2$$

$$= \frac{15}{64}$$

$$= 0.2344$$

We can also use the fact that in any probability space the probabilities add up to 1, by asking the question: What is the probability that a couple with six children will have at least two girls?

Of course, we *could* add up the values for

$$15p^4q^2 + 20p^3q^3 + 15p^2q^4 + 6pq^5 + q^6$$

But a much simpler way would be to calculate

$$p^6 + 6p^5q = \frac{1}{54} + \frac{6}{64} = 0.1094$$

and subtract it from 1, giving: $1 - 0.1094 = 0.890$.

But that way of calculating the probability of *discrete* events (we know that the events are *discrete*, even if indiscrete, because you could not have 1.75 boys and 8.25 girls!) assumes that neither p nor q are very small. The binomial distribution cannot cope with very small probabilities of random and infrequent events, unless the average rate at which they occur over given time intervals is quite large. For instance, what is the probability that lightning will strike the same boulder twice in a given year, assuming that the boulder is no different from any other boulder in the region?

Exponential growth and decay

As you know, lightning strikes are rare enough as it is, and random as well. In this way they are similar to many public health phenomena, like Marfan's syndrome or cataracts in 30-year-old women. But, due to the work of the French mathematician, Simeon Poisson (1781–1840), we now have a distribution which can handle events like this. We can apply the Poisson distribution to the frequency of random events recurring in given time intervals or in given spaces. An example of the latter would be the rate of occurrence of defective erythrocytes in a blood smear.

To understand how to use it though, we need to understand *exponential growth* and to understand that we need to remind ourselves of how compound interest works in banking. First, though, let us deal with exponents in mathematics. An *exponent* is a power, and the number raised to that power is called the *base*. Thus

$$2^5 = 2 \times 2 \times 2 \times 2 \times 2 = 32$$

The *base* of the expression is 2 and the *exponent* is 5.

If we consider an expression like 2^x, where x can equal any number (positive, negative, zero, fractional, whatever), that expression is an *exponential* expression. Exponential functions always graph as *exponential curves*. To illustrate such a curve, see Figure 8.1.

You might need reminding that, while $2^3 = 8$; $2^{-3} = \frac{1}{2^3} = \frac{1}{8}$. So no matter how negative x becomes, 2^{-x} will still always be positive, but it will *tend toward zero*, as x values further to the left of $x = 0$ are chosen.

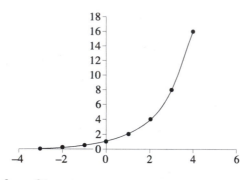

Figure 8.1 Graph of $y = 2^x$.

Natural growth and 'e'

Epidemics start off slowly. Say, each infected person infects two others, then the growth of the infection in the population will proceed for a short while like the graph of $y = 2^x$, with only positive values of x. But this will not go on for long because, as time passes and more people become infected, a *decreasing* proportion of the population affected is at risk of infection. The slope of the curve becomes less and less positive, until all of the susceptible people have become infected (*see* Figure 8.2). Notice that it is S-shaped or *sigmoid* (from the Greek *sigma*, meaning 'S').

You will see that at the heart of all natural growth is a base called 'e' (for exponential). $y = e^x$ produces a graph superficially similar to $y = 2^x$, but e does not equal 2. It is a natural constant, like π but harder to calculate. You will remember that π is that number which is always produced if you divide

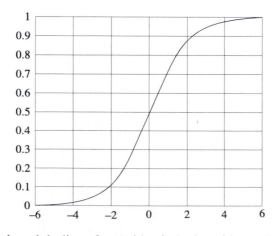

Figure 8.2 Growth and decline of an epidemic (a sigmoid curve).

any circle of *any* size by its diameter. $\pi = 3.14159$ . . . and continues on infinitely, with the decimal never becoming a repeating decimal. Likewise, $e = 2.71828$ . . . and has an infinite, never repeating decimal after the 2. But we shall prove this later.

Another example of natural growth is provided by considering the increase in body mass of a human foetus developing from one fertilised ovum. There are numerous other examples.

In trying to isolate the 'e' component in natural growth, we will have to start with a very unnatural growth phenomenon – how investments in money grow under interest in banks or building societies. There are two types of commercial interest – simple and compound. Hardly any institution uses simple interest nowadays, but suppose it did.

Your investment would grow by the same amount at the end of each *interest interval*. The *interest interval* refers to the time gap between interest payments. For instance, if you invest £100 at 10% interest *annually*, at the end of the first year you would have £110, at the end of the second year you would have £120, etc. That is, you would be adding the same amount each year.

But this growth in your money would not be curvilinear. If you wanted to withdraw your investment *halfway through* the second year, you would only get £110, not £115. On a graph, your investment growth would look like a staircase (*see* Figure 8.3).

This differs from natural growth in two respects:

1   A growing foetus does not increase its weight by an equal amount at the end of each equal time interval. It grows faster than that.
2   Over the period of its growth, it does not add to its bulk by sudden jumps, with no growth in between.

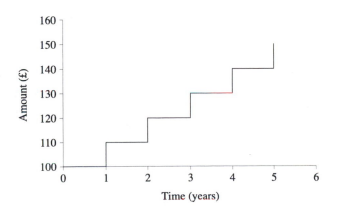

Figure 8.3 Growth of £100 invested at 10% simple interest.

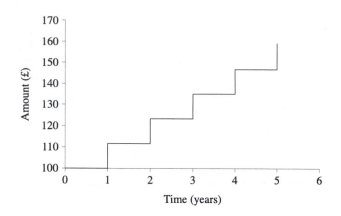

Figure 8.4 Growth of £100 over 5 years invested at 10% compound interest.

We can use our man-made system to overcome the first of these phenomena by using compound interest instead of simple interest. In compound interest, the amount to be added at the end of each interest interval is not constant, but is re-calculated each time on the basis of what is already there.

Thus, if you invested £100 at 10% compound interest per year, your investment would grow as follows. At the end of the first year you would have £110. To calculate what you would have at the end of the second year: £110 + 10% of £110 = £121. Similarly, at the end of the third year you would add on £12.10 giving you £133.10. And so on. At the end of the fourth year you would add £13.31 to £133.10 to give you £146.41 and at the end of the fifth year you would add £14.64 to £146.41 to get £161.05.

If you graphed this, you would still have a staircase pattern, but the risers would be increasing in size as you climbed the stairs! (*see* Figure 8.4).

This still doesn't look like natural growth because it grows by sudden spurts. But before we show how to solve that problem mathematically, we need to derive a general formula for compound interest.

The general formula for compound interest

The amount invested is called the principal, r% is the interest rate per annum and A is the value of your investment at any given time.

Thus, when we invested £100 for one year at 10% interest per annum, the amount after one year was

$$A = £100 + \frac{10}{100} \times 100 = 110$$

Or using the letter P for the £100

$$A = P + \frac{r}{100} \times P \text{ after one year}$$

But P is a common factor on the right hand side, so

$$A = P\left(1 + \frac{r}{100}\right)$$

Therefore, the amount at the end of year two would be given by

$$A = P\left(1 + \frac{r}{100}\right) + \frac{r}{100} \times \left[P\left(1 + \frac{r}{100}\right)\right]$$

This time, taking $P(1 + \frac{r}{100})$ out as a common factor, we have

$$A = P\left(1 + \frac{r}{100}\right)\left[1 + \frac{r}{100}\right] = P\left(1 + \frac{r}{100}\right)^2$$

In the same way, after three years

$$A = P\left(1 + \frac{r}{100}\right)^3$$

and, more generally, after q years

$$A = P\left(1 + \frac{r}{100}\right)^q$$

If the interest was rendered 4 times a year (i.e. every 3 months), the $r\%$ per annum interest every three months would be

$$\frac{1}{4} \times \frac{r}{100} = \frac{r}{400}$$

Likewise, the power of the binomial would go up by $4q$ each year and

$$A = P\left(1 + \frac{r}{400}\right)^{4q}$$

So, generalising, if the interest were rendered t times a year we would have

$$A = P\left(1 + \frac{r}{100t}\right)^{tq}$$

Changing to natural growth

In nature, of course, growth is smooth and does not proceed by sudden little jumps at the end of each interest interval. To picture that, we have to imagine the interest being rendered *an infinite number of times a year.* That is, what will be the value of A as t approaches infinity? We write this mathematically as follows

$$A = \lim_{t \to \infty} P\left(1 + \frac{r}{100t}\right)^{tq}$$

We will now simplify the argument by rearranging the formula for A, with that limit in it. First of all, the principal, P, does not vary *ever*, even as it approaches infinity. So we can write the formula like this

$$A = P \times \left[\lim_{t \to \infty}\left(1 + \frac{r}{100t}\right)^{t}\right]^{q}$$

Now, to simplify matters further, let

$$\frac{r}{100t} = \frac{1}{n}$$

$$\therefore 100t = rn$$

$$\therefore t = \frac{rn}{100}$$

So, as t approaches infinity, so does n, because $\frac{r}{100}$ is a constant.
  We can now rewrite A, using the above, as follows

$$A = P\left[\lim_{t \to \infty}\left(1 + \frac{1}{n}\right)^{t}\right]^{q}$$

That limit in the squared bracket is a constant. It is 'e' and comes out to equal 2.71828. . . . It is called the *exponential constant*. It is present in every natural growth phenomenon. We can accordingly rewrite our formula for natural growth as:

$$A = Pe^q$$

It is that e^q which makes that curve exponential, as in Figure 8.1, except that the base is not 2, but e.

Evaluating 'e'

Understanding this is not vital to public health or epidemiology but, for the curious, this is how we arrive at the value for e. It is a binomial expansion, like any other in Chapter 2, and we shall worry about the n approaching infinity as we expand, say, the first four terms. Remember the basic form. For instance

$$(a + b)^8 = a^8 + \frac{8!}{7!1!}a^7b^1 + \frac{8!}{6!2!}a^6b^2 + \frac{8!}{5!3!}a^5b^3 + \frac{8!}{4!4!}a^4b^4, \text{etc.}$$

In the same way:

$$\left(1 + \frac{1}{n}\right)^n = 1^n \frac{n!}{(n-1)!1!}(1)^{n-1}\left(\frac{1}{n}\right)^1 + \frac{n!}{(n-1)!2!}(1)^{n-2}\left(\frac{1}{n}\right)^2$$

$$+ \frac{n!}{(n-3)!3!}(1)^{n-3}\left(\frac{1}{n}\right)^3 + \dots$$

We will simplify the algebra term by term.

The first term, 1^n, equals 1.

The second term:

$$\frac{n!}{(n-1)!1!}(1)^{n-1}\left(\frac{1}{n}\right) = \frac{n(n-1)!}{(n-1)!1!} \times 1 \times \frac{1}{n}$$

$$= \frac{n}{1} \times \frac{1}{n}$$

$$= 1$$

So, the first two terms of the expression are: $1+1$.

Neither of these terms is going to be affected by n approaching infinity. Now the third term is

$$\frac{n!}{(n-2)!2!}(1)^{n-2}\left(\frac{1}{n}\right)^2 = \frac{n(n-1)(n-2)}{(n-2)!2!}(1)\left(\frac{1}{n^2}\right)$$

$$= \frac{n(n-1)}{2!n^2}$$

$$= \frac{n^2-n}{2!n^2}$$

Now we get rid of that n^2 in the denominator by dividing it into each term of the numerator, so

$$\frac{n^2-n}{2!n^2} = \frac{1-\dfrac{1}{n}}{2!}$$

So, as $n \to \infty$, $\frac{1}{n} \to 0$ and the third term becomes $\frac{1}{8!}$

Proceeding similarly with the fourth term, we get

$$\frac{n!}{(n-3)!3!}(1)^{n-3}\left(\frac{1}{n}\right)^3 = \frac{n(n-1)(n-2)(n-3)!}{(n-3)!3!} \times 1 \times \frac{1}{n^3}$$

Cancelling out the $(n-3)!$, our fourth term now becomes

$$\frac{n(n-1)(n-2)}{3!} \times \frac{1}{n^3}$$

$$= \frac{(n^2-n)(n-2)}{3!n^3}$$

$$= \frac{n^3-3n^2+2n}{3!n^2}$$

Dividing through by n^3, our fourth term becomes

$$\frac{1-\dfrac{3}{n}+\dfrac{2}{n^2}}{3!}$$

But, of course, as n approaches infinity, anything with n in the denominator approaches zero, and we are left with the fourth term equal to $\frac{1}{3!}$.

There is no need to expand and evaluate more terms because the pattern continues in the same way

$$e = 1 + 1 + \frac{1}{2!} + \frac{1}{3!} + \frac{1}{4!} + \ldots$$

Its value, to five decimal places, is: 2.71828 . . .

In natural growth, the key element will be e^x and in natural decay it will be e^{-x} (or $\frac{1}{e^x}$).

We can now go back briefly to the Poisson distribution, because in public health we frequently deal with what appear to be random outbreaks of non-contagious disease that occur unpredictably every now and then. These are a bit like the lightning strikes mentioned earlier. Kreutsfeld Jakob disease is a good example.

As pointed out in the previous chapter, *incidence* is the number of new cases of our target disease per unit time. We shall designate the *rate* of occurrence of this disease per person per unit time by the lower-case Greek letter 'lamda' or λ. Of course, the unit of time used can vary, but in public health we usually take the year as the unit of time. During epidemics, though, we frequently designate shorter intervals. During the polio epidemic of the 1940s, a week was a commonly used interval.

Using years as our time unit, we can write

$$\lambda = \frac{\text{number of new incidents}}{\text{total person-years of recording}}$$

So, if over two years, there were 68 incidents among 250 people

$$\lambda = \frac{68}{500}$$

Link between rate and risk

A healthy population is prey to a disease which is not infectious but is occurring at a rate, say, of 0.4/year. That means that 4 out of every 10 people in the population under study will acquire the disease every year. Look at Figure 8.5.

At the beginning, everyone is free of the condition, but after a year 0.4 of the population are affected and 0.6 of the population are not affected. What is

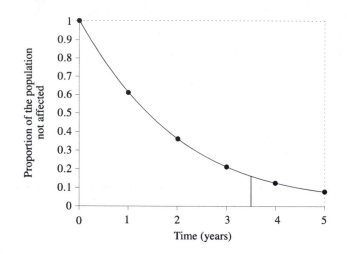

Figure 8.5 Link between rate and risk when the disease has a rate of 0.4/person/year.

important to appreciate is that, although the *rate* of the disease is great, the decline in the healthy population will not continue to decrease by the same *numbers of cases* because there are fewer unaffected people left, on which this *rate* of 0.4 can operate. So the second year *begins* with a healthy population of 0.6. Of them, 0.4 will become affected by the disease. That is, $0.4 \times 0.6 = 0.24$ will become affected. That means that by the *end* of the second year 0.64 of the population will be affected, while 0.36 will not be. During year 3, $0.4 \times 0.36 = 0.144$, so another 0.144 of the population will be stricken, making a total of 0.784 with the disease and the other 0.216 free of disease. By the end of year 4, another 0.4×0.216 of this population – namely about 0.086 – will become infected, making a total of 0.87 of the population affected and hence 0.13 free of the disease. At the end of year 5, another 0.052 of the population will be sick, making 0.92 affected and 0.08 unaffected.

Suppose we block off the part of the graph covering the first 5 years, as shown by the dotted line in Figure 8.5.

You can see that the area *below* the curve represents the proportion of the population currently *free* of the disease but *at risk* of getting it. The affected proportion of the population lies *above* this curve. If we insert a vertical bold line at, say, 3.5 years on Figure 8.5, its length will represent the proportion *at risk* of the disease *at the time.*

Our insights into exponential growth (e^x) and (e^{-x}) now allow us to apply the relevant analysis. Remembering that the *rate* is λ, it can be shown mathematically that the proportion of the population free of the disease at any time, t, is:

$$e^{-\lambda t}$$

That means that the *risk up to time t* must be

$$1 - e^{-\lambda t}$$

And the average length of time it takes to acquire the disease is $\frac{1}{\lambda}$.

If you now consider a situation in which the incidence of the disease is *very low*, say 0.02 instead of 0.4, the 'curve' will look virtually like a straight line over an interval of 5 years. Follow the calculations, doing them yourself with a pocket calculator.

At the outset, the unaffected proportion of people is 1 and the affected proportion is 0.

After	Unaffected proportion	Affected proportion
1 year	0.9800	0.02
2 years	0.9604	0.0396
3 years	0.9412	0.0588
4 years	0.9222	0.0776
5 years	0.9038	0.0960

So, even going to four decimal places it would still be indistinguishable from a straight line if you graphed it.

We can say that when λ is *very small*, the *risk* up to time t is approximately equal to λt, so that

$$\text{risk} = \lambda t$$

$$\therefore \lambda = \frac{risk}{t}$$

Poisson distribution

The foregoing now allows us to introduce the relevance of the Poisson distribution.

The Poisson distribution can be applied to analyse the rate at which an event occurs in a given time interval or over a particular space. An example of the former might refer to the number of incidents over a year of a disease among a particular population and the latter might be exemplified by analysis of a particular area of blood smear for defective erythrocytes. But Poisson analysis can only be applied *if, and only if*, the following two conditions are satisfied:

1 The events occur at random.
2 The events are independent of one another.

The second of these two criteria would seem to ordinarily rule out infectious diseases as a focus of Poisson analysis because each new event of it must have been caught from another infected person and hence not be 'independent'. However, Poisson can be so applied provided that there is not any evidence of the disease clustering. This is rather a grey area.

The Poisson distribution depends on the average number of occurrences (arithmetic mean) in a series of non-overlapping time intervals or non-overlapping areas of space. If the mean concerned is μ, the probability of n occurrences is given by

$$P = \frac{e^{-\mu}\mu^{n}}{n!}$$

Example

Two optometrists, A and B, in an NHS community hospital are trained specifically to identify early stage cataracts. To avoid waste, it is decided to get rid of optometrist B. Optometrist A sees an average of 5.1 patients per day, but *could* at a stretch handle 8. This gives him plenty of leeway and his capacity is only exceeded in 0.9 days of the year. We will say 1 day/year. If optometrist B leaves, it is estimated that optometrist A will see 7.2 patients a day. Let us use the Poisson distribution to ascertain the rate of occurrence of days/year when optometrist A's load goes beyond 8 people. Another way of putting it would be, what's the probability of optometrist A getting 9 or more patients in a one day? We do it exactly along the same lines as we do for the binomial distribution. We calculate the probability of 0, 1, 2, 3, 4, 5, 6, 7 or 8 patients /day and then subtract that from 1. This can be done with a pocket calculator with an e^{x} facility.

In each of the following calculations, we shall work out:

$$P = \frac{e^{-7.2}(7.2)^{j}}{j!}$$

For $j = 1, 2, 3, 4, 5, 6, 7$ and 8.

For $j = 1$	$P = 0.00537$
For $j = 2$	$P = 0.01936$
For $j = 3$	$P = 0.04644$
For $j = 4$	$P = 0.08359$
For $j = 5$	$P = 0.12000$
For $j = 6$	$P = 0.14458$
For $j = 7$	$P = 0.14858$
For $j = 8$	$P = 0.13373$

Therefore, we add these to get the total probabilities up to 8 patients.
Therefore, the probability of up to 8 patients = 0.70166.
Therefore, the probability that there will be 9 or more patients is

$$1.00000 - 0.70166 = 0.29834$$

In other words, for nearly a third of the time the facility will be overstretched.

Death by horse kick

In a lighter vein, let us consider a now very famous 'Health and Safety in the Workplace' application of Poisson analysis, going back to the years just after the Franco-Prussian War of 1870. The Prussian government was concerned by the number of cavalrymen injured and killed, not in battle, but by kicks from their own horses! Specifically, the number of such deaths from 1875–1894 were examined. The average number of such deaths was found to be 0.7 per year.

Therefore, the probability that no-one was killed in this way would be given by

$$P(0) = \frac{e^{-0.7}(0.7)^0}{0!} = e^{-0.7} = 0.497$$

Which means that the probability of at least one person being killed in this way in any one year was

$$1 - 0.497 = 0.503$$

The Poisson and binomial distribution compared

We said at the outset that the binomial distribution becomes increasingly insensitive as a tool the greater the difference between the probabilities of an event occurring or not occurring. The Poisson distribution, as we have seen, handles the situation of very small probabilities very well. It has its greatest applicability in situations in which we wish to determine, within a specific time-frame or physical area, what the average is of isolated, commonly infrequent, events. In such situations, the probability of the event occurring during any given time interval, or in a given area, is usually 0. But as the mean of occurrences increases, the Poisson distribution becomes less and less skewed and when the mean is 10 or more, the Poisson and the binomial distributions become virtually indistinguishable.

Chapter 9

Non-parametric statistics

What is 'non-parametric'?

All of the statistics we have considered up until now have been based on the assumption that the populations involved were normally distributed. Accordingly, we used such parameters as the mean and the standard deviation in calculations of Z, which assumed normality. Fortunately, a great many medical and biological phenomena are normally distributed. However, sometimes very little knowledge about the nature of the population is available and we cannot simply go ahead and assume that it is normal. In such cases we use *non-parametric* or *distribution-free* methods.

Just after World War II, a non-parametric test was devised by an American statistician named Frank Wilcoxon. This test is now referred to as the Wilcoxon two-sample test. It is simple and also very reliable. Since then, the use of non-parametric techniques has become widespread. As with the Student's t-test on two samples, we do have to differentiate between the situation in which the two samples are independent and the situation in which the two samples are paired (such as in two readings from each of n different patients). For the first situation, we shall consider the Wilcoxon two-sample test. For the second situation we shall consider two tests, the sign test and the Wilcoxon test for paired variates.

Wilcoxon two-independent sample test

Assume that you have two samples of size n_1 and n_2 respectively and that our H_0 is that the samples are drawn from populations having equal means. Then $n = n_1 + n_2$, where n is the total number of scores. In this test these n scores are placed in ascending order of rank. That is, for the actual data we substitute the rank-values, 1, 2, 3, . . . , n. It should be fairly obvious (think about it) that the sum of the ranks within each sample should be roughly the same if their means are equal.

However, if the total of the ranks for one of the samples is different enough from the total of ranks for the other sample, we calculate (under the assumption of equal population means) the probability of such a difference occurring by chance alone. We use the significance level, either 1% or 5%, as before, as a basis for either accepting or rejecting H_0. Let us take a real case.

Example

A new method for producing folic acid tablets has been devised. To test whether the new method has increased active-agent purity, 5 samples are made by each method with the following results:

New method: 148, 143, 138, 145, 141

Old method: 139, 136, 142, 133, 140

Has the new method increased purity? Use the 5% level of significance.

Solution

The combined data of the two samples should be arranged in increasing order of magnitude with corresponding ranks indicated, and in order to distinguish between the two samples, the variates belonging to the sample with the smaller mean are underlined. For this example, this is the sample made by the standard method.

Original data: 133, 136, 138, 139, 140, 141, 142, 143, 145, 148

Ranks: 1, 2, 3, 4, 5, 6, 7, 8, 9, 10

We now calculate the sum of the ranks corresponding to the standard method and find

$$w_1 = 1 + 2 + 4 + 5 + 7 = 19$$

while the sum of the ranks corresponding to the new method is

$$w_2 = 3 + 6 + 8 + 9 + 10 = 36$$

The total of all ranks is

$$w_1 + w_2 = 19 + 36 = 55$$

This sum, 55, is, of course, independent of the outcome of this experiment, since it represents the sum of the 10 ranks, that is $1 + 2 + 3 + \dots + 10$. If there is no effect of the new method, then the total of the ranks for the standard method, W_1 should be about the same as that for the new method, W_2. Indeed, under the hypothesis of no difference in the two methods, any sum of 5 ranks, such as $3 + 4 + 6 + 8 + 9$ would be just as likely to occur for a value of W_1 as some other sum of 5 ranks, such as $2 + 4 + 5 + 6 + 8$.

Consequently, assuming a one-tailed test, we shall now determine the probability of obtaining, among all possible sums of ranks, one which is less than or equal to the value of $w_1 = 19$ obtained in this case. This calculation is easily made: the total number of possible ways of selecting 5 ranks from 10 is the number of combinations of 10 objects taken 5 at a time, that is $C_{10,5} = 252$. Of these, the following have a sum less than or equal to 19 (note that we start by listing first the sum of ranks giving the smallest total and then proceed in a systematic way):

$$
\begin{aligned}
1+2+3+4+5 &= 15 \\
1+2+3+4+6 &= 16 \\
1+2+3+4+7 &= 17 \\
1+2+3+4+8 &= 18 \\
1+2+3+4+9 &= 19 \\
1+2+3+5+6 &= 17 \\
1+2+3+5+7 &= 18 \\
1+2+3+5+8 &= 19 \\
1+2+3+6+7 &= 19 \\
1+2+4+5+6 &= 18 \\
1+2+4+5+7 &= 19 \\
1+3+4+5+6 &= 19
\end{aligned}
$$

Consequently, since there are 12 cases, the probability of obtaining a sum of ranks less than or equal to 19 is given by

$$
P = \frac{12}{252} = 0.0477
$$

Calculation of probabilities is facilitated by use of Appendix C giving, for various sample sizes n_1 and n_2 listed in the first two columns, the corresponding values of C_{n,n_1}, where $n = n_1 + n_2$, and the number of cases for which the sum of the ranks is less than or equal to that obtained in the experiment. The column headings $0, 1, 2, \ldots, 20$ of the table represent values of the quantity

$$
U = w_1 - \frac{1}{2}n_1(n_1 + 1)
$$

Thus, if the table is used in the solution, we calculate

$$U = 19 - \frac{1}{2} \cdot 5 \cdot 6 = 4$$

Then $C_{10,5} = 252$, and the number of cases for which the sum of the ranks is less than or equal to 19 is 12, the entry in the column headed 4.

It might be of interest to note that, if the example had been solved by use of Student's t-distribution, using a one-tailed test, the probability would have been found to be $P = 0.033$. This would be the correct probability if the distribution of the population were normal. If it were not, the probability obtained by the Wilcoxon test might well be more accurate.

In the data of this example, none of the 10 given variates occurred more than once, that is, there were no ties. The question arises: How do we apply Wilcoxon's test to data with ties? The answer is supplied by Wilcoxon himself, who, when introducing his test in 1945 for the first time, gave an example in which there were several ties. This example is reproduced here. In case of ties, the procedure is the same as in the case without ties, except for the assignment of ranks.

Example

The following data give the results of fly spray tests on two preparations in terms of percentage mortality:

Sample A: 68, 68, 59, 72, 64, 67, 70, 74

Sample B: 60, 67, 61, 62, 67, 63, 56, 58

Is there a significant difference (5% level) between the two preparations?

Solution

As before, the data are arranged in increasing order of magnitude, under-lining those corresponding to the sample with the smaller mean, in this case B. Three of the variates are 67; these variates correspond to ranks 9, 10 and 11. It seems reasonable, therefore, to assign to all three of these values the mean of these ranks, namely $\frac{1}{3}$ of 30, or 10. The same procedure is followed for the two variates which are 68, corresponding to ranks 12 and 13. Again, since $12 + 13 = 25$, we assign to both variates the rank of $\frac{1}{2}(25) = 12\frac{1}{2}$. This, then, is the procedure generally followed in cases with tied data: equal ranks are assigned to tied data. For this example, then, the ranks are determined as follows:

Original data: $\underline{56}$ $\underline{58}$ 59 $\underline{60}$ $\underline{61}$ $\underline{62}$ $\underline{63}$ 64 $\underline{67}$ $\underline{67}$ 67 68 68 70 72 74

Ranks: $\underline{1}$ $\underline{2}$ 3 $\underline{4}$ $\underline{5}$ $\underline{6}$ $\underline{7}$ 8 $\underline{10}$ $\underline{10}$ 10 12.5 12.5 14 15 16

Now, since

$$w_1 = 1 + 2 + 4 + 5 + 6 + 7 + 10 + 10 = 45$$

$$U = 45 - \frac{1}{2} \cdot 8 \cdot 9 = 9$$

From the table, $C_{16,8} = 12870$, and the number of cases for which the sum of the ranks is less than or equal to 45, is 95; so that

$$P = \frac{95}{12870} = 0.00738$$

or, since a two-tailed test is needed here, the probability of obtaining a difference as great as or greater than that found between the means of the given two samples would equal

$$2P = 0.01476$$

From this we conclude that there is a significant difference between the two preparations.

The sign test for the paired case

The simplest, by far, of all non-parametric methods is the sign test, which is used to test the significance of the difference between two means in a paired experiment. It is particularly suitable when the various pairs are observed under different conditions, a case in which the assumption of normality may not hold. However, because of its simplicity, the sign test is often used even though the populations are normally distributed. In this test, as is implied by its name, only the sign of the difference between the paired variates is used. The method of applying the test will now be described.

First we determine for each pair the sign of the difference D. Under the hypothesis that the two population means are identical, the number of plus signs should approximately equal the number of minus signs. If p denotes the probability of a difference D being positive and q the probability of its being negative, we have as a hypothesis $p = \frac{1}{2}$. Suppose we are given a sample from this population and wish to determine whether it differs significantly from this hypothesis. For this purpose, we count the number of plus signs (call it S) and the number of minus signs (pairs of observations for which D = 0 are disregarded) and calculate the probability of obtaining, from a population for which $p = \frac{1}{2}$, a sample in which the number of plus signs differs as much as S or more from the expected value.

Example

In a paired experiment, the gains in weight, in pounds, of patients fed on two different diets are as given below. Is either diet superior at the 5% level of significance?

Pair	Diet A	Diet B	Sign $D = X - Y$
1	25	19	+
2	30	32	−
3	28	21	+
4	34	34	0
5	23	19	+
6	25	25	0
7	27	25	+
8	35	31	+
9	30	31	−
10	28	26	+
11	32	30	+
12	29	25	+
13	30	29	+
14	30	31	−
15	31	25	+
16	29	25	+
17	23	20	+
18	26	25	+

Solution

Disregarding the two cases where $D = 0$, we find that in the remaining sample of 16 differences 13 are positive. By means of the binomial distribution we can find the probability (under the hypothesis of equal chance for plus and minus signs) that 13 or more plus signs (or minus signs) are obtained. Since $n = 16$ is fairly large, it is convenient to use the normal curve approximation of the binomial distribution, for which

$$m = np = 8$$

$$\sigma = \sqrt{npq} = \sqrt{4} = 2$$

We need twice the area under the normal probability curve to the right of $X = 12.5$. Since

$$Z = \frac{12.5 - 8}{2} = 2.25$$

we find from the table that

$$P = 2(0.0122) = 0.0244$$

which is less than 0.05. Thus the first diet can be considered superior.

It should be noted that the sign test is applicable only if n, the number of pairs, is not too small. For example, in an experiment where $n = 5$, the probability of the most extreme case, that of all signs being either plus or minus, is $2(\frac{1}{2})^5 = 0.0625$, which is more than 5%; thus, from a sample of 5 differences, it is never possible to conclude that the hypothesis of equal population means is incorrect. Clearly then, use of the sign test at the 5% level of significance with a two-tailed test requires that n be at least 6. It should preferably be larger, and must be so if the 1% level of significance is used.

Clearly, even for a large n, we expect the sign test to have lower efficiency than the t-test, which means that in many cases the sign test will not indicate a significant difference when the t-test applied to the same problem actually shows the result to be significant. Such a situation arises if the differences corresponding to the more frequently occurring sign are large in absolute value compared with those corresponding to the other sign. Another non-parametric test which does take into consideration the magnitude of the differences and, therefore, has a higher efficiency than the sign test, is given in the next section. On the other hand, if the sign test gives a significant result, it is a valuable statistical technique requiring little calculation and, of course, no knowledge of the distribution of the population.

The Wilcoxon test for the paired case

Assume that there are given two samples whose variates are paired. In Wilcoxon's test for this paired experiment, the differences, D, for each pair are calculated and their absolute values are ranked. If there is no significant difference between the means of the two samples, then the total of the ranks corresponding to positive values of D and those corresponding to negative values of D should be about the same. If, however, the total of the ranks corresponding to one sign is appreciably less than that corresponding to the other, then, under the hypothesis of equal population means, the probability of obtaining by chance alone a sum of ranks less than or equal to w_1 is calculated, w_1 being the smaller of the rank totals. If this probability is less than the significance level, the hypothesis is rejected; otherwise, it is accepted.

Example

The data below represents counts on eight pairs of specimens, one of each specimen having received treatment A and the other treatment B.

Pair	A	B
1	209	151
2	200	168
3	177	147
4	169	161
5	159	166
6	169	163
7	187	176
8	198	188

Using the 5% level of significance, is there a significant difference between the two treatments?

Solution

Denoting the variates of the first sample by X and those of the second sample by Y, we find as follows in the table below.

X	Y	$D = X - Y$	Rank
209	151	58	8
200	168	32	7
177	147	30	6
169	161	5	1
159	166	−7	3
169	163	6	2
187	176	11	5
198	188	10	4

Note that ranks corresponding to a negative value of D are underlined; in this case, there is only one such rank, namely the rank 3, so that $w_1 = 3$. Now, under the hypothesis that there is no difference between the two treatments A and B, the probability of each difference D being positive is $\frac{1}{2}$. Consequently, the probability of obtaining any given sequence of signs for the eight differences (for example, the sequence $++-+---+$) is $(\frac{1}{2})^8 = \frac{1}{256}$, so that there are a total of 256 equally likely possibilities for the sequence of signs.

Assuming a two-tailed test, we determine the probability of obtaining among all possible sums of ranks (corresponding to negative D-values) one which is less than or equal to w_1 (in this case, 3) and then multiply this probability by 2. Now the following cases are the only ones for which the sum of the ranks (corresponding to negative D-values) is less than or equal to 3.

No negative D-value	1 case
One negative D-value with rank either 1, 2, or 3	3 cases
Two negative D-values with rank $1 + 2 = 3$	1 case
Total	5 cases

Consequently, the probability of obtaining a sum of ranks less than or equal to 3 is given by

$$P = \frac{5}{256} = 0.0195$$

and the desired probability equals

$$2P = 0.0390$$

This leads to the conclusion that the two treatments are significantly different.

Calculation of probabilities is facilitated by the use of Appendix D and Appendix E. Two tables are given for the following reason: if it is desired to find the number of cases for which the sum of ranks is less than or equal to a given value of w_1, where w_1 is less than or equal to n, then this number of cases is independent of n and the table in Appendix D can be used. This was true in the previous example, where $w_1 = 3$ and $n = 8$. For this example, Appendix D shows the number of cases for which w_1 is less than or equal to 3 to be 5.

If, however, it is desired to find the number of cases for which the sum of ranks is less than or equal to a given value of w_1, where w_1 is greater than n, then this number of cases depends on n and Appendix E must be used.

The chi-square test

Probably the most famous of all the non-parametric tests – so famous, in fact, that a lot of people don't even realise it is non-parametric – is the chi-square test. The Greek letter 'chi' is our χ and so the test is described in writing as the χ^2 test.

This test is used in a situation in which you know ahead of time what values you should get (your 'expected' values) and with which you can then compare the results you actually did get (your 'observed' values). For instance if you cross a heterozygously black guinea pig with a homozygously white guinea pig, simple Mendelian genetics would lead you to be believe that $\frac{3}{4}$ of the resulting young should be black and $\frac{1}{4}$ of them white. Thus, if the guinea pig produced a litter of 24, then 18 should be black and 6 should be white. Your expected (E) values should be 18 and 6. But in actual fact, the guinea pig (being ignorant of both Mendelian genetics and statistics) produced 15 black and 9 white; these are your observed (O) values.

We use the χ^2 formula, which is

$$\chi^2 = \sum_{i=1}^{n} \frac{(E_i - O_i)^2}{E_i}$$

In our case, it is

$$\chi^2 = \sum_{i=1}^{2} \frac{(E_i - O_i)^2}{E_i}$$

$$= \frac{(18 - 15)^2}{18} + \frac{(6 - 9)^2}{6}$$

$$= \frac{9}{18} + \frac{9}{6}$$

$$= \frac{36}{18}$$

$$= 2$$

What you actually do with that value of χ^2, and what it means, will be explained as applied to a number of uses to which χ^2 can be put. First follow through these various 'cases', then we shall consider how to actually calculate and interpret chi-squared scores.

One-sample case

A lecturer in anatomy wanted to ascertain whether a set of student exam scores was distributed normally.

If there were a range of scores from 40 to 90 and a large enough number of subjects, the scores could be allocated to intervals of 5 points: 40–44, 45–49, 50–54, etc. The frequencies of scores actually falling within each of these categories would be counted. Then he would have to work out how many scores should theoretically fall into each interval on the basis of the normal distribution. This would require him to work out the proportion of area under the curve in each interval so that he could multiply this in each case by the total number of scores to obtain the required theoretical values. He would then use the χ^2 test to see if his observed scores deviated significantly from the theoretical ones. If on carrying out this test, he obtained a significant χ^2 score, then he could conclude that his obtained scores did deviate significantly from normality.

Thus we see that the χ^2 test produces a value reflecting the deviation of observed values from expected or theoretical values. In the example given in the previous paragraph, if the observed number in each interval had been identical with the number expected to fall in each interval under the normal distribution, then the χ^2 value would obviously have been zero. So it is clear that the greater the difference between observed and expected frequencies, the larger the value of χ^2 becomes and hence more likely that it is significant.

The χ^2 table (Appendix I) will be explained in greater detail in working an actual problem in a subsequent section of this chapter, but we can say that each χ^2 value is interpreted according to the number of degrees of freedom in the particular analysis. In a one-sample test, such as the one just described, the number of degrees of freedom is the number of categories, or cells, less one. In the case of the examination scores just discussed, each of the intervals would be a cell. There are ten such intervals between 40 and 90, hence 9 degrees of freedom.

It must not be thought that the χ^2 one-sample test can be used only with respect to comparison with the normal distribution. It can be used whenever a result is to be compared with an expected ratio or any other arbitrarily defined distribution.

Suppose, for instance, that a clinician wishes to know whether a new method of treating second degree burns resulted in new tissue formation within 24 hours in more cases than did a previously well-established treatment. Under the old system, 22% of treated patients generated new tissue within 24 hours whereas 78% did not. On the new treatment, say, 35 patients out of 92 did regenerate new tissue in the first 24 hours while the rest did not. In this case the theoretical ratio was 22:78. Thus under theoretical conditions, the ratio for 92 patients would be $(0.22 \times 92) : (0.78 \times 92)$ or 20:72. We must compare that with 35:57.

A case of two unrelated samples

The test can be used when the measures in the samples are only nominal. The actual calculation of χ^2, after the data have been distributed in their categories and a frequency count taken, proceeds almost as described earlier for the one-sample case. The fundamental difference is that we do not need to calculate theoretical frequencies from some arbitrary model but directly from the data in hand.

Suppose that we wished to determine whether children who come from homes where no musical instrument is played by a member of the family performed any differently on a tone-perception test than did children from 'musical' homes. The tone perception test was only a two-way test – either the subject could discriminate or they could not. Out of 200 people taking the tone test, 100 came from 'non-musical' homes and 100 came from 'muscial' homes. The results of the test are presented below.

	Passed	*Failed*	*Total*
Musical homes	80	20	100
Non-musical homes	40	60	100
Total	120	80	200

In this case, the theoretical values are rather easy to calculate. We are assuming as our null hypothesis, H_0, that there is no significant correlation between tone perception and opportunity to hear a family member practising a musical instrument. Therefore, since half come from non-musical homes, then we would expect that the passes and fails on the tone perception test should be divided evenly between the two categories of children. So of the 120 who passed, we should *theoretically* expect (if H_0 is true) that 60 came from musical homes and 60 from non-musical homes. Similarly, we would expect 40 of the failures to come from musical homes and 40 to come from non-musical homes.

As the previous χ^2 test explained, χ^2 in this case depends on the magnitude of the deviations of expected from observed values in each of the categories. If χ^2 is large enough to be significant according to the table, then that would indicate that the disparity between theoretical and observed values is so great that it is unreasonable to continue to believe H_0.

More than two unrelated samples

As we have seen, chi-square can be used with nominal-type data (so long as frequencies are assigned to the different categories specified). We have also seen that it can be used to test the difference between an actual sample and some hypothetical distribution, and also to test differences between two or more actual examples. Very few alternatives to chi-square exist for testing data that is nominal.

The fundamental equation for χ^2 is given as follows

$$\chi^2 = \sum_{i=1}^{n} \frac{(O_i - E_i)^2}{E_i}$$

where O_i are the observed values, E_i are the expected values and n is the number of values. The reader must note the following rule very closely and be sure to take account of it in carrying out calculations. Whenever χ^2 is calculated from 1×2, or 2×2 tables, an adjustment known as Yates correction for continuity must be used. This involves subtracting 0.5 from the absolute value (ignoring the + or − sign) of the numerator before it is squared on each χ^2 calculation. Since the formula above must be calculated for each cell and then all of these values be added up, it would make some difference to the final χ^2 value if the Yates correction were carelessly forgotten.

Thus, for the cases involving 1×2, or 2×2 tabular displays we have

$$\chi^2 = \sum_{i=1}^{n} \frac{(|O_i - E_i| - \frac{1}{2})^2}{E_i}$$

Three problems involving χ^2 will now be carried out in full.

Problem 1

A sociologist is faced with the data shown below, and he wishes to ascertain if the figures for 1970 differ significantly from figures for the previous ten years. The people in social classes A and B are from the same street.

	Social class A	Social class B
Number of felony convictions for 1970	45	15
Percentage of felony convictions 1957–69	40	60

Solution

He has observed data on 60 cases from the two social classes concerned in a given neighbourhood. Of these 60 people, he could *expect* 40% (or 24 of them) to be to be from social class A and 36 of them to be from social class B.

$$\chi^2 = \frac{(|45 - 24| - \frac{1}{2})^2}{24} + \frac{(|15 - 36| - \frac{1}{2})^2}{36}$$

$$= 17.5 + 11.7$$

$$= 29.2$$

Notice that this was a 1×2 table, so the Yates correction for continuity was used. In using the χ^2 table to see if our computed value was significant, we have to know the number of degrees of freedom to use – for a one-sample case, the number of cells less one. Since there are only two cells in this case, the number of degrees of freedom is 1. We now look up the chi-square table in Appendix I and observe that with one degree of freedom a χ^2 value equal to or greater than 3.84 is needed to reject the null hypothesis at the 0.05 level of significance, while at the 0.01 level of significance, a value equal to or greater than 6.64 is sufficient to reject H_0. Since our computed value is 29.2, we can certainly reject H_0, even at the 0.01 level of significance.

That means that the sociologist is justified in believing that some new factor has entered the picture, causing social class A people to be convicted more often than before and/or causing social class B people to be convicted less often than before. After carrying out this test and obtaining a result like this, he might begin an investigation into the reasons behind this significant change in conviction patterns.

Problem 2

This problem illustrates the use of chi-square in handling differences between two samples. A test of attitude toward a certain political question was administered to 100 soldiers who had voluntered to serve and to 100 soldiers who had been conscripted. The data obtained were as shown below.

	Agree	Neutral	Disagree	Total
Volunteers	40	40	20	100
Conscripts	60	20	20	100
Total	100	60	40	200

Do a chi-square test to see if volunteers differ significantly from conscripted soldiers with respect to the question concerned.

Solution

There are an equal number of conscripts and volunteers, so of the 100 who agree we would *expect* 50 from each category, of the 60 who were neutral we would *expect* 30 in each category and of the 40 who disagree we would *expect* 20 in each category – if H_0 is to be upheld. Our calculation of χ^2, then, should look as follows*

$$\chi^2 = \frac{(40 - 50)^2}{50} + \frac{(40 - 30)^2}{30} + \frac{(20 - 20)^2}{20} +$$

$$\frac{(60 - 50)^2}{50} + \frac{(20 - 30)^2}{30} + \frac{(20 - 20)^2}{20}$$

$$= 2.0 + 3.3 + 0 + 2.0 + 3.3 + 0$$

$$= 10.6$$

For two or more samples, the degrees of freedom necessary to use the chi-square table is equal to the number of rows minus one times the number of columns minus one, which is $(2 - 1)(3 - 1) = 2$.

With 2 degrees of freedom, the χ^2 table tells us that at the 0.01 level, values equal to or in excess of 9.210 are significant. Since our computed value is 10.6, our results are significant and we reject H_0.

A word should be said here about the number of cells it is advisable to have in using chi-square. In general, the larger the number of cells or categories, the more sensitive will be the χ^2 test – so the more categories that we can have, the better. but if when working out the expected values, some cells have fewer than 5 in them as an expected frequency, that invalidates the test. That is, it does not matter if fewer than 5 are *observed* in a given category, as long as 5 or more are *expected* in each category. Now the question arises as to what to do if it happens that after an experimenter has set out his categories, his expected frequencies violate the rule in some categories.

In that case, we reduce the number of categories until the frequencies expected in each category exceed five. For instance, in an attitude test like the one discussed in Problem 2, there might have been five original choices for

---

* We do not need the Yates correction for continuity here because the tabular array is 3×2, not 1×2 or 2×2.

each question, namely: strongly agree, agree, neutral, disagree, strongly disagree. Then, when the expected values were calculated, it turned out that there were fewer than five in some cells, the number of categories would be reduced by combing 'strongly disagree' with 'agree' and 'disagree' with 'strongly disagree'.

Problem 3

We shall now present and solve a problem involving more than two samples. In a plastics factory employing 1200 people there are three departments: moulding, tinting and assembling. The company psychologists have worked out about how many people from each department can be expected to have been absent in a year for the following periods: never, 1–3 days, 4–6 days, a week or more. In the data that follows the psychologists' figures are presented in parentheses, while the actual absence figures are given without parentheses. We wish to compare the two sets of figures.

Department	Never	1–3 days	4–6 days	A week or more	Total
Moulding	400 (400)	100 (87.5)	50 (50)	50 (62.5)	600
Tinting	300 (266.6)	50 (58.3)	25 (33.3)	25 (41.7)	400
Assembling	100 (133.3)	25 (29.2)	25 (16.7)	50 (20.8)	200
Total	800	175	100	125	1200

Now the reader may wonder how the expected frequencies were calculated by the psychologists. This is important and we shall illustrate how it is done by considering the expected frequency of the upper right corner cell. You take the proportion between the first row total and the total (which is $\frac{600}{1200}$ and multiply that by the fourth column total (125)). This gives

$$125 \times \frac{600}{1200} = 62.5$$

Solution

The χ^2 value is now worked out as follows

$$\chi^2 = \frac{(400 - 400)^2}{400} + \frac{(100 - 87.5)^2}{87.5} + \frac{(50 - 50)^2}{50} +$$

$$\frac{(50 - 62.5)^2}{62.5} + \frac{(300 - 266.6)^2}{266.6} + \frac{(50 - 58.3)^2}{58.3} +$$

$$\frac{(25 - 33.3)^2}{33.3} + \frac{(25 - 441.7)^2}{41.7} + \frac{(100 - 133.3)^2}{133.3} +$$

$$\frac{(25 - 29.2)^2}{29.2} + \frac{(25 - 16.7)^2}{16.7} + \frac{(50 - 20.8)^2}{20.8}$$

$$= 0 + 1.79 + 0 + 2.50 + 4.16 + 1.18 +$$

$$2.07 + 6.69 + 8.32 + 0.60 + 4.13 + 40.99$$

$$= 72.43$$

The number of degrees of freedom involved is the number of rows less one multiplied by the number of columns less one. That gives $(4 - 1)(3 - 1) = 6$ degrees of freedom. Even at the 0.001 level of significance, the value we have obtained is significant – as discovered by using the chi-square table in the usual way.

Study exercises 6

1 The measurements of the heights (in inches) of six adults of each of two different nationalities are given below

> Nationality A: 64, 67, 68, 65, 62, 61
>
> Nationality B: 69, 70, 66, 63, 71, 72

Use Wilcoxon's two-sample test to determine whether there is a significant difference in mean heights for these two nationalities (5% level).

2 In an experiment consisting of 25 pairs, the number of plus signs exceeds the number of minus signs. If a two-tailed test is applied, how many minus signs can there be, at most, to allow us to consider the results significant on the basis of the 5% level of significance?

3 In a paired feeding experiment, the gains in weight (in pounds) of subjects fed on two different diets are as listed below. Can either diet be considered superior at the 5% level of significance? (Use the Wilcoxon test.)

Pair	Diet A	Diet B
1	27	19
2	30	32
3	31	21
4	34	33
5	23	27
6	31	34
7	39	34
8	34	28
9	33	26
10	35	26

Chapter 10

For the algebraically innocent

Measuring correlations

We often notice, in medical work, that two sets of measurements seem to be 'related'. For instance, pyrexia and pulse rate are often related – the higher the fever, the higher the pulse rate. Likewise, severity of cystitis and urine flow are usually related. The more positive the degree of cystitis (however measured), the more scanty (usually) is the urine flow.

Such relationships are obviously of very great importance in analysing disease states. For instance, it is not always true that establishing that every time a variable A increases variable B also increases, means that A causes B (or vice versa). They might both be related to a third variable, for instance. But in statistics we do have ways of investigating such relations, or lack of them, with a useful degree of precision. Unfortunately, although the reasoning is simple enough, it does require that the student has a ready grasp of elementary algebra. This chapter, then, is written for those who do not believe that they are so equipped. The phenomena that this chapter will allow you to understand and use, and which is concerned with the whole business of the 'relatedness' or otherwise of variables, is called 'correlation'.

Straight line equations

You are no doubt aware that any algebraic statement, such as $x^2 + 4y = 7$ or $x = 6 + 2y$, etc. can be converted to a visual representation on a plane surface called a graph. It is also important to realise that any such graph likewise can be expressed in terms of algebra – so that you have a one-to-one correspondence between them. Any given algebraic statement (called an 'equation' if an equal sign is involved) corresponds with one and only one shape of graph, and any given shape of graph corresponds with one and only one algebraic representation of it. Naturally, this does not take the use of different variables into account, so that clearly

$$4xy^3 - 3x^2 + 9y$$

is the same algebraic representation as

$$4pq^3 - 3p^2 + 9q$$

Let us look briefly at how we move from the algebra to the picture.

Locating points

Every point on a plane can be uniquely located by an ordered pair of numbers, provided we have agreed as to what specific point represents $(0, 0)$. We do this by what are called Cartesian coordinates, named after the French philosopher René Descartes, who first worked out the idea.

Let the 'y-axis' be a vertical straight line (also called the ordinate) and the 'x-axis' be a horizontal straight line (called the abscissa). The point at which they cross, thus dividing the plane into 4 quadrants, is referred to as $(0, 0)$ – at that point $x = 0$ and $y = 0$. The point $(0, 0)$ is also known as the 'origin'. As you move along the x-axis to the right of $(0, 0)$ the x-values become increasingly positive and as you move along it to the left of $(0, 0)$ they

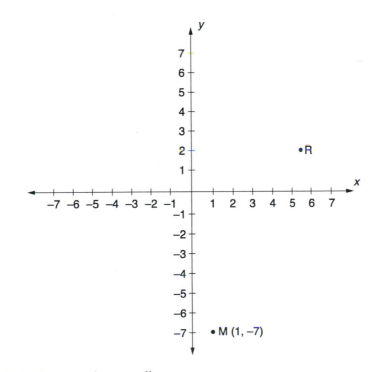

Figure 10.1 The Cartesian coordinates.

become increasingly negative. Likewise, with the y-axis. As you move from $(0, 0)$ up the y-axis, the values become increasingly positive and as you move down the y-axis below $(0, 0)$ the values become increasingly negative. Thus, to locate a point, M at $(1, -7)$ in Figure 10.1, say, we do it in exactly the same way we would on a map. The first value is always the horizontal component (the x-value) and the second value is always the vertical component (the y-value). So in the case of the point M we go 1 unit to the right on the x-axis, then 7 units straight down.

In exactly the same way, we can specify the locaton of some existing point, such as R in the diagram. The coordinates of R are $(5\frac{1}{2}, 2)$ because we get to it by going $5\frac{1}{2}$ units to the right of the origin and 2 units up.

Graphing algebraic expressions

In our treatment of correlation, we shall only be interested in straight line or 'linear' graphs. Let us first try to go from the algebraic equation, say $3x - 5y = 9$, to its graph. To 'graph' it we can pick any value for one of the variables and solve for the other one. That will tell us the coordinate of one of the points through which the line passes. You probably appreciate that any two distinct points through which a straight line passes are all you need to be able to draw it. For that reason, we do the same thing again, using a different value, to get the coordinates of a second point through which the line represented by $3x - 5y = 9$ passes. Then we can graph it. Enough theory, let us actually do it!

Before that, though, you must appreciate that an algebraic equation of a straight line represents a line of infinite length. So, unless it is exactly parallel with the x-axis or with the y-axis, it does pass through a point somewhere on its route where $x = 5891$, say. That is, for any x, there will be a corresponding y. Not being masochists, we pick much easier values to work with.

Let $x = 1$. Then $3x - 5y = 9$ becomes

$$3 - 5y = 9$$

so

$$-6 = 5y$$

so

$$y = -\frac{6}{5} = -1.2$$

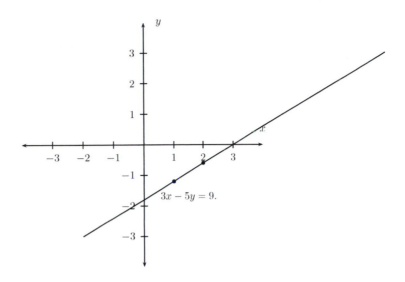

Figure 10.2 The graph of $3x - 5y = 9$, drawn using the points $(1, -1.2)$ and $(2, -0.6)$.

This means that our line passes through the point $(1, -1.2)$. Of course, that is not enough information to allow us to graph it, for an infinite number of straight lines pass through that point. OK. Let $x = 2$. Then $3x - 5y = 9$ becomes

$$6 - 5y = 9$$

$$-5y = 3$$

$$y = -\frac{3}{5}$$

$$= -0.6$$

So a second point through which our straight line passes is $(2, -0.6)$. Two distinct points are all we need to completely determine a straight line. See the diagram in Figure 10.2. We can do it even more simply by finding out what the y-value is when $x = 0$ and what the x-value is when $y = 0$. These two values, to which we will make constant reference in talking about correlation, are called the y-*intercept* and the x-*intercept*, respectively.

Let's do it to $3x - 5y = 9$.

If $x = 0$, then $y = \frac{9}{5} = -1.8$ and if $y = 0$, then $x = 3$.

You see, by using 0 values we did not even have to do much written calculation. You can figure them in your head.

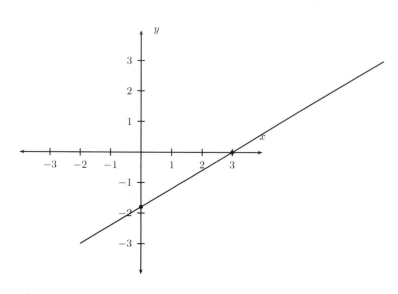

Figure 10.3 The graph of $3x - 5y = 9$, drawn using the points $(0, -1.8)$ and $(3, 0)$.

Now, draw the graph. The two points are $(0, -1.8)$ and $(3, 0)$. Make sure you get those pairs in the right order – that's why they are called ordered pairs. Notice two things. We see from Figure 10.3 that the graph is identical to that for the points $(1, -1.2)$ and $(2, -0.6)$ because the same equation is being graphed in both cases, and secondly, by substituting in 0 for x then 0 for y, we see the x and y intercepts immediately. The x-intercept is $+3$ (where the line cuts or intercepts the x-axis) and the y-intercept is -1.8 (where the line cuts or intercepts the y-axis).

One question must have crossed your mind in all this: we have said that, unless a straight line is exactly parallel with either the x-axis or the y-axis, it will pass through every x-value (with a corresponding y-value) or every y-value (with a corresponding x-value). But how do you know if it is parallel, say, to the x-axis: it will never cross it and thus everywhere on the line will have the same y-value. Thus: $y = -5$ is a straight line parallel with the x-axis and 5 units below it. In the same way: $3x = 2$ is a straight line parallel with the y-axis and $\frac{2}{3}$ of a unit to the right of it. So, if you see a straight line equation in which only one variable is named, then it is referring to a line parallel to one of the axes.

Ah, I hear you ask, how do you tell whether a given algebraic equation is a straight line equation or not? It is a straight line equation if neither the x nor the y (or whatever the two variables might be – there's no law saying they have to be x and y) are raised to a higher power than one. Thus: $2x + 7y = 3$ is a straight line, but $4x^2 - 5y = 1$ is going to be a curve, as would $x^2 + y^2 = 6$ or even $7 = 5xy$.

Straight lines and their gradients

Every straight line has a *gradient* or *slope*. For the purpose of our discussion, let's use the word 'slope'. The *slope* of a straight line tells you two things:

- whether the line slants up as you move from left to right, or slants down as you move from left to right along it
- how steeply it rises or falls as you move from right to left along it.

Slope, designated by the letter 'm' in mathematics, is measured by the ratio

$$m = \frac{rise}{run}$$

Thus, if for every 6 units of horizontal displacement to the right, a straight line moves up 5 units, we say

$$m = \frac{5}{6}$$

Note that the numerator of the fraction refers to the *vertical* displacement (the rise) and the denominator refers to the *horizontal* displacement (the run). If for every 4 units a line moved to the right, it *dropped* 7 units, then its slope would be given by

$$m = -\frac{7}{4}$$

So the sign of the slope tells you right away which way the line is slanting and the fraction itself tells you how steeply.

It should be obvious, even for the algebraically naïve, that if the line is straight its slope is constant for any distance on it. Thus, if a line rises 5 units for every 2 units of horizontal displacement to the right, then it will rise $7\frac{1}{2}$ units for 3 units horizontal displacement to the right, and it will drop $12\frac{1}{2}$ units for every 5 units horizontal displacement to the left.

Calculating a straight line's slope

There are several ways of doing this. If we know the coordinates of two distinct points on the line, the matter is very simple. Suppose we know that it passes through (8, −1) and (5, 9). First, let's put those two points in horizontal order from left to right. Surely $(8, -1)$ is to the right of $(5, 9)$ because the x-value 8 is larger than the x-value 5. We list them, then

$$(5, 9) \text{ and } (8, -1)$$

The horizontal displacement from $x = 5$ to $x = 8$ is obviously 3. $8 - 5 = 3$. Over that displacement, the line drops (which means its slope is negative) from $y = 9$ to $y = -1$, a total of 10 units. That is, it goes from 9 units above the x-axis to 1 unit below the x-axis. $9 - (-1) = 10$.

So its slope is given by

$$m = -\frac{10}{3}$$

A very steep line indeed. I'd hate to cycle down that one!

Suppose a straight line passes through the point $(-5, 2)$ but we don't know anything else about it, we can give a general formula for its slope by nominating any other point on the line as being, say, (x, y). Then

$$m = \frac{y - 2}{x - (-5)} = \frac{y - 2}{x + 5}$$

That idea will come in useful later.

Suppose we are just given the equation of the straight line and nothing else. Can we work out its slope? Yes, indeed. Watch and concentrate.

You know that, from the equation alone, we can work out the x and y intercepts. But that gives us the coordinates of two points on the line and, as we have just seen, we can easily work out the slope given the coordinates of two points through which the line passes.

Look. Consider the equation

$$3x = 4 - 11y$$

You realise, of course, that there are several legal ways of writing it

$$3x + 11y = 4$$
$$y = -\frac{3}{11}x + \frac{4}{11}$$
$$x = -\frac{11}{3}y + \frac{4}{3}$$

etc.

Whichever way we write it, if $x = 0$, the $y = \frac{4}{11}$, and if $y = 0$, then $x = \frac{4}{3}$. So the y-intercept is $\frac{4}{11}$ and the x-intercept is $\frac{4}{3}$.

Keep those two intercepts in mind. We will come back to them in a few moments. In any case, they immediately provide us with the coordinates of the two points through which our line passes. They are

$$\left(0, \frac{4}{11}\right) \quad \text{and} \quad \left(\frac{4}{3}, 0\right)$$

That means the run (horizontal displacement) is $\frac{4}{3}$ (or $\frac{4}{3} - 0$) and the rise (vertical displacement) is $-\frac{4}{11}$ (or $0 - \frac{4}{11}$). Thus, the slope of our line is given by

$$m = \frac{-\dfrac{4}{11}}{\dfrac{4}{3}} = -\frac{4}{11} \times \frac{3}{4} = -\frac{3}{11}$$

Without using the minus sign in our calculation, we can tell that the slope is going to be negative, because, as we move to the right from $x = 0$ to $x = \frac{4}{3}$, the line drops from $y = \frac{4}{11}$ to $y = 0$.

Now there is one more really interesting and vital feature of all this. Remember that the slope is $-\frac{3}{11}$ and you will see something most gratifying.

Let us rewrite the equation to begin with $y = \ldots$.

The original equation was $3x + 11y = 4$. We can express that as

$$11y = -3x + 4$$

But that can be written as

$$y = -\frac{3}{11}x + \frac{4}{11}$$

Do you notice anything? Remember, $-\frac{3}{11}$ is our slope and remember also that $\frac{4}{11}$ is our y-intercept. That means that a straight line equation, if written in terms of $y = \ldots$, will take the form

$$y = mx + b$$

where b is the y-intercept and, of course, m is the slope. Hence, simply by rewriting any straight line equation, we can find the slope of that line.

Example

What is the slope of

$$5p + 2q - 20 = 0$$

Solution

We can transform it in stages, if your algebra is a bit shaky

$$5p + 2q = 20$$

$$2q = -5p + 20$$

$$q = -\frac{5}{2}p + 10$$

So if q is taken as the vertical axis and p as the horizontal axis, the line slants down as we move from left to right along it. Its slope is $-\frac{5}{2}$ and it cuts the q-axis 10 units above the origin.

Going from graph to algebra

One last thing we need to consider before moving on to correlation is how to go from the 'picture' to the equation. Often we have graphed data and wish to express it in terms of an algebraic equation to communicate the results more effectively, or even to predict with them.

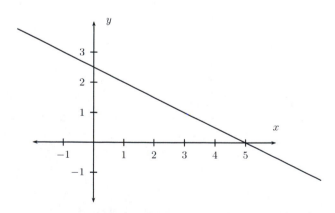

Figure 10.4 The graph with unknown equation.

Let's try it with the graph in Figure 10.4. Well, the y-intercept is $2\frac{1}{2}$ or $\frac{5}{2}$ and the x-intercept is 5. Therefore, two points through which the line passes are

$$(5,0) \quad \text{and} \quad \left(0, \frac{5}{2}\right)$$

The slope, clearly negative, therefore is given by

$$m = \frac{\frac{5}{2}}{-5} = -\frac{5}{10} = -\frac{1}{2}$$

If we now use the slope-intercept form

$$y = mx + b$$

where $m = -\frac{1}{2}$ and $b = \frac{5}{2}$, we get

$$y = -\frac{x}{2} + \frac{5}{2}$$

Therefore, our equation can be written

$$2y + x = 5$$

If your algebra is sufficiently weak, either through having forgotten it since doing it (sins of comission) or having never met it before (sins of omission), that you have had to read this chapter, really make sure you understand it before ploughing on. The Study exercises which follow are designed to give you a good strong basis for going on.

Study exercises 7

1   Which of the following equations are straight line equations:
   (a) $4x - 7y + 5 = 0$
   (b) $m^2 + 2p = 6$
   (c) $kl^5 = 8$
   (d) $x = \frac{5}{9}$
   (e) $p = 4q + 2$
2   Write each pair of points in order from left to right:
   (a) $R = (-2, 1)$, $S = (-7, -4)$

(b) $K = (-5, -19)$, $L = (-3, 2)$
(c) $P = (0, 6)$, $Q = (-1, 6)$
(d) $A = (2, 0)$, $B = (3, 0)$
(e) $X = (1, 9)$, $Y = (1, 7)$

3 Find the slopes of the line segments joining the points in No. 2, as follows:
(a) SR
(b) KL
(c) QP
(d) AB
(e) XY

4 Change each equation to the form

$$y = mx + b$$

which is the 'slope-intercept form' and then write its slope and y-intercept.
(a) $4y - 2x + 5 = 0$
(b) $3s + t = 9$
(c) $\frac{2}{3}k - \frac{4}{5}l - 2 = 0$

5 Write the equation of the straight line which passes through the point $(5, -2)$ and for which the slope is $\frac{1}{3}$.

6 Write the equation of the straight line which has a y-intercept of 2 and an x-intercept of -3.

Chapter 11

The Gini coefficient

The non-clinical context of health

In the heroic battle of public health against disease, it is easy to become so
pre-occupied with the medical aspect that we forget that, globally speaking,
the leading cause of ill-health is poverty. Therefore, those of us concerned
with global health frequently have to analyse the distribution of incomes,
both within individual nations and between nations. An increasingly
used statistical tool in this is the Gini coefficient, and it makes use of the
Lorenz curve. For that reason, today's research workers and students of
epidemiology and public health will frequently see Gini coefficients cited.
The following will enable such people to understand them.

The Lorenz curve explained

The Lorenz curve is a graph that shows, for the lowest x% of households (the
abscissa measure on the graph), what percentage the corresponding y% (the
ordinate measure on graph), of the population have, consider Figure 11.1.

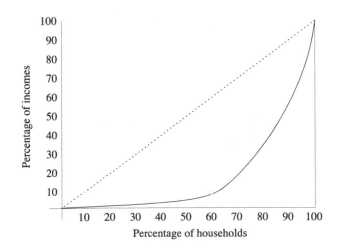

Figure 11.1 A Lorenz curve of income distribution of a hypothetical population.

In the population shown in Figure 11.1, the increases are very unfairly distributed.

For instance, 50% of the households account for only 40% of the income! Even 80% of the households account for only 40% of the income! The broken straight line, running at a 45° angle to the x-axis and having a positive slope, on the other hand, would represent a perfectly fair distribution, because the more the curve deviates from the straight line of slope +1, the less fair the distribution is.

It was Max O Lorenz, a US economist, who developed the curve that takes his name, in 1905. An Italian statistician, by the name of Corrado Gini, carried Lorenz's work just that bit further to give us the Gini coefficient, which allows us to make better analytic comparisons. The Gini coefficient is a vital tool in discussing human rights and it is important for the reader to at least appreciate how it works.

The Gini coefficient

Originally intended to systematise and more rigorously quantify Max O Lorenz's analysis of unequal income distributions, the Gini coefficient can be used to analyse any form of uneven distribution. The Gini coefficient is a number between 0 and 1, when 0 corresponds to 'perfect equality'. In other words, it allows us to calculate a measure of the degree to which a distribution deviates from the 'perfect', which is represented by the broken line in Figure 11.2, below.

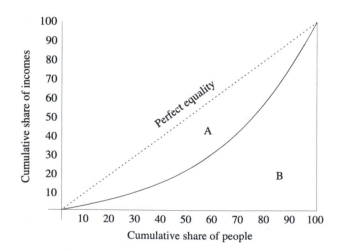

Figure 11.2 Graph for calculating a Gini coefficient.

In a state of perfect equality, the Gini coefficient would equal 0, and in a state of complete inequality, where one person in the community in the population had all the income, the Gini coefficient would equal 1. Figure 11.2 represents neither of these. But how do you calculate the Gini coefficient?

Notice that in Figure 11.2 we have designated the area between the Lorenz curve and the perfect equality line as A. Likewise, the area between the x-axis (abscissa) and the Lorenz curve is designated B. Then the Gini coefficient, G, is given by the formula:

$$G = \frac{A}{A + B}$$

The reader will find that, in some publications, the G-score is multiplied by 100, so those scores can range from 0 to 100 instead of from 0 to 1. Although no hard and fast rule prevails, this practice seems to be increasing.

Using this formula will introduce a slight inaccuracy because of some rather involved statistical phenomena arising, which control variance, using the formula characteristics of G. However, this problem is overcome by multiplying the value you get for G by the fraction $n/n+1$, where n is the number of individuals (or communities) used.

Calculation of the areas A and B does require integral calculus. But a more practical formula is given by

$$G = 1 - \sum_{K=1}^{n}(X_K - X_{K=1})(Y_K + Y_{K-1})$$

The use of the capital Greek letter Σ, called 'sigma', means to sum up the areas of all the 'rectangles', each represented by each particular value of

$$(X_K - X_{K=1})(Y_K + Y_{K-1})$$

for any given value of K. Sigma notation used in such calculations is explained fully in the author's *Foundations of Mathematical Analysis* book.[1] Remember though that, in some presentations, the Gini score is multiplied by 100, so that the scores range from 0 to 200 instead of from 0 to 1.

Gini coefficients worldwide

Tables 11.1 and 11.2 show how Gini indices allow us to compare countries by income inequality. These values are derived from *Gap Between Rich and Poor: World Income Inequality*.[2]

Table 11.1 Thirty countries with the greatest inequality

	Country	Gini index	Lowest 20%	Highest 20%
1	Sierra Leone	62.9	1.1%	63.4%
2	Central African Republic	61.3	2.0	65.0
3	Swaziland	60.9	2.7	64.4
4	Brazil	60.7	2.2	64.1
5	Nicaragua	60.3	2.3	63.6
6	South Africa	59.3	2.9	64.8
7	Paraguay	57.7	1.9	60.7
8	Colombia	57.1	3.0	60.9
9	Chile	56.7	3.3	61.0
10	Honduras	56.3	2.2	59.4
11	Guinea-Bissau	56.2	2.1	58.9
12	Lesotho	56.0	2.8	60.1
13	Guatemala	55.8	3.8	60.6
14	Burkina Fasso	55.1	4.6	60.4
15	Mexico	53.1	3.5	57.4
16	Zambia	52.6	3.3	56.6
17	Hong Kong, China	52.2	4.4	57.1
18	El Salvador	52.2	3.3	56.4
19	Papua New Guinea	50.9	4.5	56.5
20	Nigeria	50.6	4.4	55.7
21	Mali	50.5	4.6	56.2
22	Niger	50.5	2.6	53.3
23	Gambia	50.2	4.0	55.3
24	Zimbabwe	50.1	4.7	56.7
25	Venezuela	49.5	3.0	53.2
26	Malaysia	49.2	4.4	54.3
27	Russia	48.7	4.4	53.7
28	Panama	48.5	3.6	52.8
29	Cameroon	47.7	4.6	53.1
30	Dominican Republic	47.4	5.1	53.3

Table 11.2 Thirty countries with the greatest equality

	Country	Gini index	Lowest 20%	Highest 20%
1	Slovakia	19.5	11.9%	31.4%
2	Belarus	21.7	11.4	33.3
3	Hungary	24.4	10.0	34.4
4	Denmark	27.4	9.6	34.5
5	Japan	24.9	10.6	35.7
6	Sweden	25.0	9.6	34.5
7	Czech Republic	25.4	10.3	35.9
8	Finland	25.6	10.0	35.8
9	Norway	25.8	9.7	35.8
10	Bulgaria	26.4	10.1	36.8
11	Luxembourg	26.9	9.4	36.5
12	Italy	27.3	8.7	36.3
13	Slovenia	28.4	9.1	37.7
14	Belgium	28.7	5.3	37.3
15	Egypt	28.9	9.8	39.0
16	Rwanda	28.9	9.7	39.1
17	Croatia	29.0	8.8	38.0
18	Ukraine	29.0	8.8	37.8
19	Germany	39.0	8.2	38.5
20	Austria	31.0	6.9	38.0
21	Romania	31.1	8.0	39.5
22	Pakistan	31.2	9.5	41.1
23	Canada	31.5	7.5	39.3
24	Korea, South	31.6	7.5	39.3
25	Poland	31.6	7.8	39.7
26	Indonesia	31.7	9.0	41.1
27	Latvia	32.4	7.6	40.3
28	Lithuania	32.4	7.8	40.3
29	Spain	32.5	7.5	40.3
30	Netherlands	32.5	7.3	40.1

From Tables 11.1 and 11.2 the reader can see immediately the difference between the developed and less developed countries. For, instance, most European nations have Gini coefficients ranging between 0.24 and 0.36. The US is markedly further away from income equality and since 1985 has been above 0.4. In this way, human rights activists and scholars can quantify the debate with respect to welfare policies. But, as we shall see later, the Gini coefficient can lead us astray if we try to use it to make glib political comparisons between large and much smaller countries (e.g. US and Cuba). Let us consider, say, Hungary and Denmark. These two countries have the lowest *G*-values in the EU. They were calculated separately in drawing up Tables 11.1 and 11.2. But in the US all the states (of course) are calculated together, despite the fact that California, for instance, is extraordinarily rich, while some of the US states rate with less developed countries. If each US state is calculated separately, their *G*-score will generally be lower than those calculated for the country as a whole.

In the US, as elsewhere, we see considerable variations of *G*-scores over time. See Table 11.3 below. But we note that it is increasing, suggesting greater internal inequity.

Strengths of *G* as a measure of income inequality

1 Measures such as the Gross Domestic Product (GDP) are not good measures for inter-country comparison because GDP is skewed by extreme values, meaning that a GDP may well be very unrepresentative of most people in the country. The *G*-score has a big advantage because it measures degrees of inequality, rather than an average.
2 The *G*-score can be compared across countries and is easy to interpret. By comparison, GDP calculations are cumbersome and insensitive to variations across a given population.
3 We can use *G*-scores to compare income distributions between various communities in a national population. As we would expect, for instance, *G*-scores between urban and rural areas within one country usually differ

Table 11.3 Changes in US *G*-score over 30 years

Year	G-score
1970	0.394
1980	0.403
1990	0.428
2000	0.462

markedly. When extremes of wealth and poverty are widely characteristic of both urban and rural sub-populations (as in the US), the rural and urban *G*-score will remain close.

4 Because *G*-scores seem to vary over time, they are useful in indicating how income distribution has changed over time in any one country.

5 *G*-scores are independent of the size of the economy being measured. The same is true for population size differences.

Critical comments on the use of *G*-score

1 As we have already seen with the US, if we use the Gini coefficient over a geographically large and diverse nation it will tend to result in a larger score than if the sub-regions are calculated individually. This, for example, makes it rather meaningless to compare the *G*-scores of individual EU nations with that of the US as a whole.

2 Comparing incomes from country to country on the basis of *G*-scores is problematical because countries can have widely different welfare systems. For instance, a nation which provides housing and/or food stamps to its less fortunate citizens, will have a higher G-score than some which don't because vouchers do not count as income using Gini.

3 Even if two nations have the same Gini coefficient, they may still differ greatly as far as income distribution is concerned. For instance, suppose that in nation A, half the households had no income and the other half · shared the entire income equally, it will have a Gini of 0.5. But so will nation B in which the dictator has the entire nation's income and everyone else is equal – with no income at all!

4 Statistically speaking, the Gini coefficient responds more sensitively to incomes in the middle of the range than to incomes at the extremes.

These problems, especially the last one, have led to extra tests or variations on Gini being elaborated. One of these is the 'Hoover Index', also known as 'Robin Hood'. It is equal to that portion of the total income that would have to be redistributed for there to be perfect equality. The reader can think of it as the longest vertical distance between the Lorenz curve which, remember, is the cumulative portion of the total income held below a certain income percentile, and the straight line of slope + 1. Hoover indices are often used in establishing links, within a society, between socio-economic status (SES) and health.

Another one commonly referred to is the Atkinson Index. It is one of the few that is actually biased, intentionally, to the poorer end of the spectrum so that it can be used in making judgements about the efficacy or otherwise of welfare programmes. It is derived by calculating what Atkins called the 'equity–sensitive average income', designated 'ye', and which is defined as that level of per capita income which – if enjoyed by everyone – would bring about total welfare equal to the total welfare generated by actual income distribution. The calculation of 'ye' is itself complex because it involves calculation of a so-called 'inequality aversion parameter' or 'E' requiring rather esoteric mathematics. However, those details are not necessary for the reader to appreciate the argument. The E reflects the strength of a society's preference for equality and can take values ranging from zero to infinity. When E is greater than 0, there is a social preference for equality. As E increases in value, society attaches more weight to income transfers at the lower end of the distribution, while attaching less weight to such transfers at the upper end of the distribution.

The actual Atkinson Index (1) is given by the formula

$$I = 1 - \frac{ye}{m}$$

where 'm' is the mean income of the population. The more equal the income generation, the closer 'ye' will be to 'm' and thus the lower will be the Atkinson Index. I values range between 0 and I.

References

1 MacDonald T. *Foundations of Mathematical Analysis.* Delhi: Ajanta Books; 2005.
2 World Development Index. *Gap Between Rich and Poor: World Income Inequality.* Washington: The World Bank; 2006.

Chapter 12

Correlation: a measure of relatedness

Are they cor-related or co-related?

Until now we have been considering only single variable distributions, such as height, IQ, etc. and how to describe statistics associated with them. However, two variables (such as depression states and memory) are often inter-related and we wish to discover how, whether one causes the other or whether they tend to be directly or inversely related, etc. In pure sciences, such as chemistry and physics, relations between variables are often perfect or very nearly so. This is rarely the case in the social sciences. Where human behaviour is concerned it would be difficult to think of a case in which one could realistically exclude the operation of all but two variables or even define perfectly the variables over which we have no control.

The technique used to describe the magnitude and direction of the relation between two or more variables is called *correlation*. One measure that statisticians commonly use to describe the degree of the relation of one variable to another is called the Pearson product-moment correlation coefficient, and this is designated '*r*'.

But before we go into the details, can you account for why the spelling of this statistical phenomenon should be 'correlation' and not 'corelation'?

If two variables are related in such a way that they both change in the same direction, for instance, measures of eyesight and scores in rifle school during military training, the variables are said to be positively correlated. If two such variables change in opposite directions, such as scores on various anxiety scales and social adaptability, their correlation is said to be negative.

The coefficient of correlation ranges from -1.00 through 0 to $+1.00$. An *r*-value of 1 is perfect positive correlation (such as the relation between heights measured in centimetres and heights measured in inches), while an *r*-value of -1 indicates perfect negative correlation.

Consider the following data. Ten patients are each given two respiratory efficiency tests, X and Y. The pairs of scores are shown below.

Student	X	Y
A	41	53
B	38	48
C	36	45
D	33	44
E	29	40
F	26	36
G	25	36
H	20	31
I	19	28
J	15	26

We can put this bivariate (two variables) data on a graph as in Figure 12.1. A glance at the graph will indicate that although the correlation between X and Y scores is not perfect, they certainly seem to be roughly positively correlated because the higher the X scores the higher (usually) are the associated Y scores. This is an example of an approximately linear correlation. There are bivariate distributions in which the two variables are correlated but in a way which can best be approximately described by a curve of some kind rather than a line. However, in this book we shall concern ourselves entirely with linear correlation and shall not consider curvilinear correlation.

Computing a value for correlation

Let us begin the task of computing r by considering it in terms of deviations from the mean for each variable. To simplify this discussion we must introduce another notation. Until now whenever we have mentioned, say, X we have thought of it in terms of one item of data. We shall now begin to think of X, and of any other we choose to use as a variable, in two ways:

- X, as a capital letter, to stand for one measurement, one data item
- x, as a small letter, to mean $X - \bar{X}$.

For the data that we were given in the previous section, we can calculate $\bar{X}$ and $\bar{Y}$ and find all the x-scores and all the y-scores by subtracting $\bar{X}$ from each X entry and $\bar{Y}$ from each Y entry. See the table on p. 151.

The reader should now ponder the following important point. By subtracting the appropriate mean from each score in each variable, we have, in effect, subtracted a constant value from each score. Therefore, the scatter diagram of the deviation scores will not be different in shape from the scatter diagram of the original score. This is because adding or subtracting a constant from a score does not change the relative position of the scores

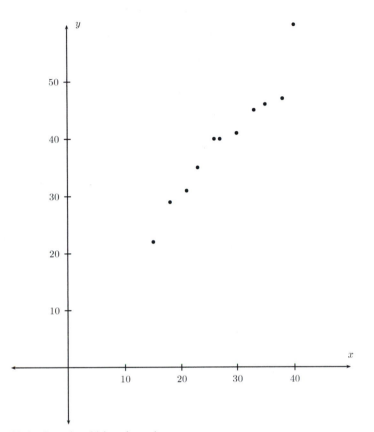

Figure 12.1 Graph of bivariate data.

but only the location of the scores on the scale used. If the reader is doubtful about this statement he should consult Figure 12.2, where the scatter diagram of the deviation scores is displayed.

Student	X	Y	x	y
A	41	53	12.8	14.3
B	38	48	9.8	9.3
C	36	45	7.8	6.3
D	33	44	4.8	5.3
E	29	40	0.8	1.3
F	26	36	−2.2	−2.7
G	25	36	−3.2	−2.7
H	20	31	−8.2	−7.7
I	19	28	−9.2	−10.7
J	15	26	−13.2	−12.7
	$\bar{X} = 28.2$	$\bar{Y} = 38.7$		

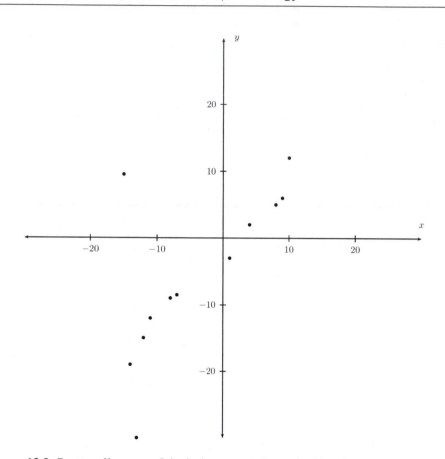

Figure 12.2 Scatter diagram of deviation scores from the bivariate data.

Now for each student, suppose we multiply the two deviation scores and then add all of the products. What would the final sum tell us? Think carefully as we answer this question. The reader might have to go over this section several times. Consider three cases.

1 If the scores are positively correlated, then they both change in the same direction. Thus a large positive x-score will be associated with a large positive y-score and their product will be a large positive number. Similarly, a large negative x-score will be associated with a large negative y-score and their product will also be a large *positive* number because the product of two negatives is positive. In the same way, each product will give a positive number, but decreasing in magnitude as the individual deviation scores become numerically smaller. If either x or y is zero then the associated product will be zero, but provided that the scores are positively correlated there will be no (or very few) negative products xy.

Thus the *sum* of all of the *xy*-values in that case will be a large positive number.

2   If the scores are negatively correlated, then they change in *opposite* directions. Thus associated with a large positive *x* is a large negative *y*, and vice versa. So it can be seen that, even as the numerical values of the *x*'s and *y*'s get smaller, their signs will generally be different and hence their products negative. Thus the sum of all of the products *xy* will be a large negative number if the scores are negatively correlated.

3   If the scores are not correlated at all, then the sum of the products *xy* will be equal to zero, or be numerically small at any rate. This is because some positive *x*'s will be associated with positive *y*'s and some with negative *y*'s, and likewise with negative *x*'s, so that some of the products will be negative and some positive. In summing them, the negative and positive values will tend to cancel one another out.

We can use a notation that we already know to simplify this account radically – namely the sigma notation for summation. In this case we have been discussing

$$S = \sum_{i=1}^{n} x_i y_i$$

where *i* runs from 1 to 10 if there are 10 pairs. Thus *S* can be thought of as a measure of correlation (or lack of it) because:

- if *S* is very large and positive, the scores are positively correlated
- if *S* is very large and negative, the scores are negatively correlated
- if *S* is at or close to zero, the scores are not linearly correlated to any great degree (although they might be curvilinearly correlated).

However, *S* is not a very satisfactory measure of correlation because there is nothing implicit in it that can guide us in deciding what is to be meant by very large positive or very large negative. For instance, we might be measuring *X* (increase in temperature in 0.1 degrees Celsius) and *Y* (increase in weight in milligrams of amoeba in a culture). At any rate, the actual numbers in *X* and *Y* would be very small, so that even a perfect positive correlation might result in *S* = 0.06, or something like that. Moreover, even given those conditions, that same measure of correlation would increase in value according to the number of pairs of scores, whatever the degree of correlation or otherwise of the variables. By the same token, the number of kilograms of asphalt laid daily on all the roads in Australia (*X*) is not very highly correlated with the daily death toll due to disease in India (*Y*), yet for these two variables *S* is almost bound to be quite large numerically, either negatively or positively, because the individual values of X and Y (and hence x and y) are so very large.

Therefore we have to have some form of maintaining the advantage in terms of *sign* that $\sum xy$ gives us as a measure of correlation without letting the actual *size* of the measure be influenced by extraneous factors that have nothing to do with the actual *degree* of correlation between two variables.

The Pearson product-moment correlation coefficient

The variation in numerical size of $\sum xy$ according to these extraneous factors can be eliminated by dividing $\sum xy$ by $ns_x s_y$, where s_x refers to the standard deviation of the X-variable and s_y refers to the standard deviation of the Y-values. This has been proven in mathematics, but the argument is too involved to consider here. Thus the expression

$$\frac{\sum_{i=1}^{n} x_i y_i}{ns_x s_y}$$

is a valid measure of correlation. It is called the Pearson product-moment correlation coefficient and is designated r. So we have a few formulae to make use of

$$r = \frac{\sum_{i=1}^{n} x_i y_i}{ns_x s_y}$$

n, of course, indicates the number of pairs entering into the calculation. A variation of this formula is

$$\frac{\sum_{i=1}^{n} Z_{x_i} Z_{y_i}}{n}$$

where $Z_{x_i} Z_{y_i}$ is the product of the Z-score for the ith X-value and the Z-score for the associated i^{th} Y-value. Again, this equivalence can be rather easily proven in mathematics, but there is little point in doing so in a book of this nature. Finally, the most convenient calculational formula for 'r', although it would be a nightmare to memorise is

$$r = \frac{n\sum_{i=1}^{n} X_i Y_i ash; \sum_{i=1}^{n} X_i \sum_{i=1}^{n} Y_i}{\sqrt{\left(n\sum_{i=1}^{n} X_i^2 - \left(\sum_{i=1}^{n} X_i\right)^2\right)\left(n\sum_{i=1}^{n} Y_i^2 - \left(\sum_{i=1}^{n} Y_i\right)^2\right)}}$$

Now, the real advantage of 'r' is that it can only range between -1 and $+1$ and thus can give us an indication of the relative magnitude of a correlation, whatever the magnitude of the measurements being considered. Thus, $r = +0.9$ would be more positively correlated than $+0.2$.

How about remembering formulae?

In another section we shall deal with the formula for r if the data is grouped. However, a word must be said at this point about the use and misuse of statistical formulae.

Formulae are certainly economical print-wise. Imagine expressing the technique for calculating r by means of words alone. Moreover, providing one is reasonably alert with respect to very elementary algebra, formulae are far less ambiguous than prose is likely to be. Formulae confer a level of precision which words rarely do.

Having said that, though, this author must reiterate a point made in the preface which is that there is little to be gained by memorising complicated formulae such as those for r. We find it worthwhile to memorise simple basic formulae, such as those for the mean or for standard deviation, because they clearly reflect fundamental definitions which we need to use to reason with statistical material. The various formulae for r also, of course, reflect definitions and basic ideas, but only via an involved chain of sophisticated mathematical argument. If the reader has not made use of and understood the mathematical argument used in deriving such formulae, then of what intellectual value is it for him to memorise the result, because he certainly cannot think with it? It might be argued that the user of statistics should even memorise results of which he does not understand the derivation in case he has to use them, but that is a poor argument. In real life, if a social scientist (or anyone else) wishes to use a complicated statistical formula, he can look it up in a text.

The important thing to know, if one wishes to become an efficient user of statistics, is what weapons are available in the statistician's arsenal, how to use them and under what circumstances. Memorising formulae does not expedite that.

Using the value r

Consider the data shown on page 151, just below Figure 12.1, let us calculate r from it

$$\Sigma X = 282$$

$$\Sigma X^2 = 8638$$

$$\Sigma Y = 387$$

$$\Sigma Y^2 = 15687$$

$$\Sigma XY = 11607$$

$$n = 10$$

So

$$r = \frac{(10)(11607) - (282)(387)}{\sqrt{((10)(8638) - (282)^2)((10)(15687) - (387)^2)}}$$

Thus

$$r = \frac{116070 - 109134}{\sqrt{(86380 - 79524)(156870 - 149769)}}$$

$$= \frac{6936}{\sqrt{(6858)(7101)}}$$

$$= \frac{6936}{(82.8)(84.3)}$$

$$= 0.9937$$

This would seem to indicate a very high degree of positive correlation. We must, however, be cautious of using r scores loosely in coming to conclusions, as the reader will come to realise in subsequent discussion in this chapter.

Calculating *r* from grouped data

In this discussion we shall be making use of data from Figure 12.3, but not all at one time. Therefore, the reader should not be frightened off on first glancing at Figure 12.3. It is a truly horrifying sight to behold, but if he carefully reads this section he will see how easily it falls into place from what he already knows.

The scatter diagram shows the joint distribution of two variables: IQ (X) and anatomy (Y). Just informally from the tally marks, one would judge that r is positive in this case. The reader will notice that there are 50 tally marks and that each such mark is determined by two scores (one X and one Y).

In the lower left of the table, the letters A to F have been used to identify the six *rows* at the bottom of the table. The letters A to F at the upper right of the table identify the six *columns* at the right of the scatter diagram. The reader should be absolutely clear that he understands the difference between row and column in this context. A row is a horizontal arrangement of elements. A column is a vertical arrangement of elements.

- The frequency of scores within each IQ score interval can be read from row A (F_X), by which we notice, for instance that the IQ score interval with the highest frequency is (116–119).
- Row B and column B list, repectively, d_X and d_Y, which are deviations from an arbitrary origin divided by the interval size. The arbitrary origin of anatomy scores is at (25–29).
- The entries in row C ($f_X d_X$) and column C ($f_Y d_Y$) are obtained by multiplying each f_X by its corresponding d_X and each f_Y by its corresponding d_Y.
- The entries in row E (Σd_Y) are obtained in the following way: within each column of the scatter diagram, add up the d_Y values of the tally marks. For example, the fourth entry from the left in row E, 35, is the sum of d_Y values

$$(3 \times 4) + (3 \times 5) + (1 \times 8) = 35$$

Score	88–91	92–95	96–99	100–103	104–107	108–111	112–115	116–119	120–123	124–127	128–131	132–135	136–139	140–143	A f_Y	B d_Y	C $f_Y d_Y$	D $f_Y d^2_Y$	E Σd_X	F $d_{XY}\Sigma d_X$
100–104										I					1	15	15	225	9	135
95–99								I	I	I					3	14	42	588	24	336
90–94							I		I			I			3	13	39	507	25	325
85–89							I		II					I	4	12	48	576	35	420
80–84										I	I	II			4	11	44	484	41	451
75–79						I	II	II			I				6	10	60	600	41	410
70–74								II							2	9	18	162	14	126
65–69				I											1	8	8	64	3	24
60–64					II	II			I						5	7	35	245	26	182
55–59					II	II									4	6	24	144	18	108
50–54				III	I			II		I					7	5	35	175	37	185
45–49				III				I							4	4	16	64	16	64
40–44		I			I				I						3	3	9	27	13	39
35–39															0	2	0	0	0	0
30–34	I	I													2	1	2	2	1	1
25–29														I	1	0	0	0	13	0
															50		395	3863	316	2806
A f_X	1	2	0	7	6	5	4	8	6	3	3	3	0	2	50					
B d_X	0	1	2	3	4	5	6	7	8	9	10	11	12	13						
C $f_X d_X$	0	2	0	21	24	25	24	56	48	27	30	33	0	26	316					
D $f_X d^2_X$	0	2	0	63	144	125	144	392	384	243	300	363	0	338	2450					
E Σd_Y	1	4	0	35	36	37	36	77	57	40	26	35	0	12	395					
F $d_X \Sigma d_Y$	0	4	0	105	140	185	216	539	456	360	260	385	0	156	2806					

Figure 12.3 Correlation of grouped gata.

So the fourth Σd_Y entry in row E is 35. Similarly, column E (Σd_X) entries are obtained.

- Row F and column F entries are clearly obtained by multiplying each Σd_Y entry by its corresponding d_X and each Σd_X entry by its corresponding d_Y.

When data are grouped, our formula for r becomes

$$r = \frac{n\Sigma(d_Y d_X) - (\Sigma f_X d_X)(\Sigma f_Y d_Y)}{\sqrt{n\Sigma f_X d_X^2 - (\Sigma f_X d_X)^2}\sqrt{n\Sigma f_Y d_Y^2 - (\Sigma f_Y d_Y)^2}}$$

Using this now on the data in our table, we obtain

$$r = \frac{(50)(2806) - (316)(395)}{\sqrt{(50)(2450) - (316)^2}\sqrt{(50)(3863) - (395)^2}}$$

$$= \frac{15480}{\sqrt{22644}\sqrt{37125}}$$

$$= \frac{15480}{(150.48)(192.68)}$$

$$= 0.53$$

Remarks about *r*

We can say that an r-value is a convenient *index* of relationship but that it is not proportional, necessarily, to the degree of relationship. It is common for instance, to speak loosely of r-values as being 'high' or 'low' without adequate reference to the type of data to which they refer. Coefficients of correlation as high as 0.5 between measures of a physical and mental trait are so rare that an r-value in this context of 0.6 would be regarded as incredibly high. On the other hand, an r-value of 0.9 between two mental traits (say, two tests of reading comprehension) would be regarded as only medium or low, especially if the tests were thorough.

Another mistake commonly made is to assume that an r-score can tell us something about cause and effect. It cannot be validly argued, for example, that because a high correlation exists between measures of reading comprehension and arithmetic ability, arithmetic ability is therefore dependent upon reading comprehension or vice versa. It may be true of course, but it does not follow from the statistical evidence of correlation. Correlation between variables may be due to a third factor, or set of factors, entirely unrelated to the other two.

For instance, height is usually directly related to age in children, as is reading ability. We would therefore expect reading ability and height to be positively correlated without one having caused the other.

Any interpretation on cause and effect relationships must be based upon logical considerations of the nature of the variables. A correlation coefficient by itself can give no definite information about it.

The sampling distribution of *r*-scores

Suppose a population (bivariate) has a correlation *r*, at or near 0.0, then large samples taken from it will have *r*'s that are distributed roughly normally. However, if *r* is close to either end of the *r*-scale, say near −1.0, then the sample *r*'s will not be normally distributed due to the crowding effect of the fixed boundaries on *r*. The distribution of sample *r*'s in this case will be very much positively skewed, as shown in Figure 12.4. A British statistician by the name of RA Fisher, however, worked out a method of transforming sample *r*-scores so that the distribution of these transformed scores was normal. Therefore, whenever we wish to work with sampling *r*'s, we first transform them to their appropriate Fisher transformation values (called *Z*) and then work with those. Any answers that we thus derive will be in terms of *Z*-scores and thus must be transformed back if we wish to speak of our results in terms of *r*.

A table (*see* Appendix G – Fisher *Z*-transformations) has been worked out enabling us to convert *r*-scores to *Z*-scores for this purpose of using sampling *r*'s. The *Z* coefficients, as we have said, are distributed normally regardless of the *r*-values or the size of the sample. The standard error of *Z* is given by

$$SE = \frac{1}{\sqrt{n - 3}}$$

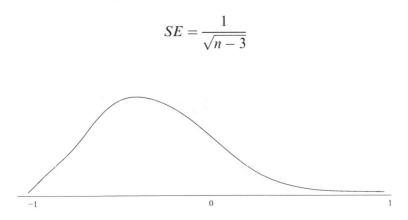

Figure 12.4 Sampling distribution of *r*'s when $r = 0.1$.

That is, σ_Z depends only on n and not on r. For instance, suppose we had a sample of 84 with an r-value of 0.61. Therefore

$$SE_Z = \frac{1}{\sqrt{n-3}} = \frac{1}{\sqrt{81}} = \frac{1}{9} = 0.111$$

Now for an r of 0.61 we look up the corresponding Z coefficient in the Fisher transformation table and find that an r of 0.61 corresponds to $Z = 0.71$.

Let us use this information to obtain the confidence interval at the 0.95 level (*see* Figure 12.5). $Z = 1.96$ for a probability of 0.025, therefore

$$\frac{Z - 0.71}{0.111} = 1.96$$

so

$$Z = (1.96)(0.111) + 0.71 = 0.218 + 0.71$$

So the upper value of the 0.95 confidence limits on Z is $0.71 + 0.218 = 0.928$. The lower value is thus given by $0.71 - 0.218 = 0.492$. Therefore, our 0.95 confidence limit on a Z coefficient of 0.71 is (0.492, 0.928).

To make this information usable to us, though, we have to remember to translate it back to r-scores by using the Fisher transformation table backwards. We find that a Z coefficient of 0.492 is associated with an r-value of 0.455, while a Z coefficient of 0.928 is associated with an r-value of 0.730. So the 0.95 confidence limit on $r = 0.61$ is (0.455, 0.730).

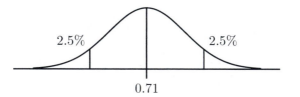

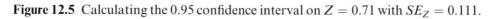

Figure 12.5 Calculating the 0.95 confidence interval on $Z = 0.71$ with $SE_Z = 0.111$.

Chapter 13

The problem of prediction

Linear correlation

Suppose that in a bivariate distribution, two variables are linearly correlated. Even if they are not perfectly related in this way, the reader can see that a straight line graph could be drawn which represents the relationship more closely than any other straight line.

For instance, consider the scatter diagram of bivariate data in Figure 13.1. Superimposed on the scatter diagram are three straight lines, L_1, L_2 and L_3. Any one of these, or even some other one, might be selected as an approximation of the relationship between X and Y, but the reader can see that neither L_1 nor L_3 is a very good approximation. L_2 on the other hand, is a pretty good approximation.

It is convenient to have such an approximate straight line graph once a linear relation between two variables has been demonstrated. This is so because for a given value of X (one of the variables) it is possible to predict the associated value of Y (the other variable) when neither the given X nor its associated Y are actually presented in the data at hand. A glance at Figure 13.2 will make this clear.

Suppose the X-value indicated is not listed in the data given and we wish to predict what Y-value would be associated with that X-value. We would go along the X-axis and find the relevant X-value and then measure the vertical distance (in terms of the Y-scale) from that point to the prediction line. That distance would then be our predicted Y-value. L is the prediction line. In psychology and medicine there are many applications of this. For instance, IQ scores (X) are linearly correlated with reading comprehension (Y). An appropriate prediction line graph has been drawn. A teacher has in her class a boy with IQ 133 and she wants, for any one of several reasons, to be able to predict his level of reading comprehension. Therefore, she finds the value of 133 on the IQ axis and from that measure the vertical distance to the prediction line in terms of units on the reading comprehension scale. This measure is then the value she is looking for.

In real life, of course, there are tables for such well-known correlations, but the example given should enable the reader to understand the theory behind the problem.

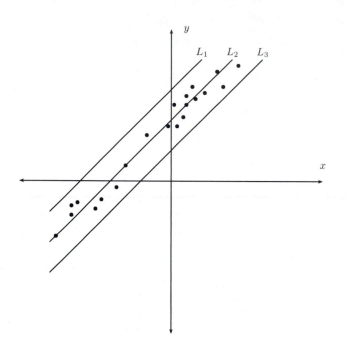

Figure 13.1 Scatter diagram of bivariate data.

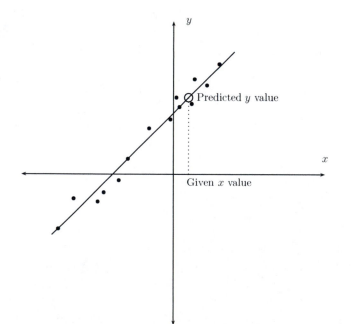

Figure 13.2 Predicting Y from X.

Back to the algebra

Now the algebra to which you were so rudely introduced in Chapter 10 can come to your assistance, especially the slope-intercept form of a straight line equation.

To make use of these mathematical facts in a bivariate situation in which you have made some measure of it (by finding the r-coefficient), we use two important formulae, one giving the slope of the prediction line and one giving the Y-intercept or b-value. With these two numbers, we can then write the prediction equation and proceed to use it.

For rather interesting historical reasons, the prediction line used in this statistical context is usually called the *regression line*.

Remember that the regression line only gives us an estimate of Y, indicated by $\hat{Y}$. The regression line is the line which best fits the data, but unless the data is absolutely linear, even the regression line cannot be a perfect fit. Where our regression line is given by

$$\hat{Y} = mX + b$$

the two formulae we need are

$$m = \frac{n\Sigma XY - (\Sigma X)(\Sigma Y)}{n\Sigma X^2 - (\Sigma X)^2}$$

and

$$b = \bar{Y} - m\bar{X}$$

Thus, m must be calculated *first* because the value of m is needed to work out b.

Suppose that we have established that IQ and reading comprehension are approximately linearly related and we wish to find the regression (prediction) line for predicting reading comprehension scores from IQ scores. How would we do it using the data in the table below?

Student	IQ (X)	Reading (Y)
A	126	82
B	109	77
C	111	77
D	124	95
E	133	80
F	107	44
G	122	87
H	101	53

$$\Sigma X = 933$$

$$\Sigma X^2 = 109677$$

$$\Sigma XY = 70367$$

$$\Sigma Y = 595$$

$$\Sigma Y^2 = 46321$$

In order to carry out this calculation, you would have to add three more columns to the table: a column for X^2 values, a column for Y^2 values and a column containing XY-values with one XY-value for each pair.

Therefore

$$m = \frac{(8)(70367) - (933)(595)}{(8)(109677) - (933)^2}$$

$$= \frac{562936 - 555135}{877416 - 870489}$$

$$= \frac{7801}{6927}$$

$$= 1.13$$

Now

$$b = \bar{Y} - m\bar{X}$$

$$= \frac{595}{8} - (1.13)\frac{933}{8}$$

$$= 74.38 - 131.79$$

$$= -57.41$$

Therefore, our regression equation is

$$\hat{Y} = 1.13X - 57.41$$

Hence, what reading comprehension score would you predict for a student with an IQ of 120?

$$\hat{Y} = 1.13(120) - 57.41 = 78.19$$

So, we could predict a reading comprehension score of 78.19. Two other commonly used formulae for the slope of the regression line are

$$m = r\frac{S_Y}{S_X}$$

and

$$m = \frac{\Sigma XY}{\Sigma X^2}$$

The first of these two formulae is rather useful in medical statistics, because you almost surely will have calculated r *before* trying to establish the regression line.

Where to from here?

In the last two chapters, you have been introduced to the two very important phenomena of correlation and prediction, but on the basis of a non-rigorous explanation in which lots of mathematical justification has been omitted. The purpose in this, as in the entire book, is to enable you to be able to decide rationally whether or not your particular research needs call for the calculation of r and its application to a linear correlation equation. Such insight, of course, will not confer competency in actually carrying out the task. The best way, by far, of gaining that competency is to actually generate data to which it is appropriate to apply these statistical procedures. As an aid to the acquisition of competency, though, especially if your particular health work does not involve appropriate data at the moment, two 'problems' are given in the study exercises which follow. The second one involves no calculation, so how can this help you to acquire competency? Answer this question to youself first, before you address the other two!

Study exercises 8

Subject	X	Y
1	7	20
2	32	2
3	13	16
4	9	19
5	20	15
6	13	15
7	24	2
8	23	4
9	13	14

1 Tests X and Y were administered to the same nine subjects with the results in the table above.
   (a) Calculate r_{XY}.
   (b) What is S_Y?
   (c) What proportion of the variance in X is associated with variance in Y?
2 Doctors found, in the sixties, a positive correlation between smoking and lung cancer and concluded that smoking caused lung cancer. Fisher commented acidly, between puffs, that lung cancer caused smoking. Suggest a plausible third explanantion.

Chapter 14

Introducing ANOVA

What can ANOVA do for you?

Analysis of variance, abbreviated ANOVA, is of cardinal importance in statistical work involving data from the health sciences. The reader must appreciate that this chapter is merely an introduction to the topic and is designed to familiarise them with the concept and to equip them to carry out very simple analyses of variance.

We have already considered techniques for studying the differences between means of samples to see if we can ascertain, within the limits of probability, whether or not the difference is significant at some pre-arranged level of significance (α). If it is, then we conclude that the second sample differed so much from the first that it is highly unlikely that they came from the same population to begin with. Now analysis of variance was developed to help solve the following sort of situation.

Suppose that instead of having only two different treatments, to each of which we expose a sample and then test the differences between their means, we have six different treatments to each of which a sample has been exposed. For the sake of argument, let the six treatments be A, B, C, D, E and F and let the means of the six associated samples be $\bar{X}_A$, $\bar{X}_B$, $\bar{X}_C$, $\bar{X}_D$, $\bar{X}_E$ and $\bar{X}_F$. If we now want to see if one or more of these means differs significantly from any other, we would have only one way of doing it with what we already know. We would have to compare $\bar{X}_A$ with $\bar{X}_B$, $\bar{X}_A$ with $\bar{X}_C$, $\bar{X}_A$ with $\bar{X}_D$, $\bar{X}_A$ with $\bar{X}_D$, $\bar{X}_A$ with $\bar{X}_E$, $\bar{X}_A$ with $\bar{X}_F$, $\bar{X}_B$ with $\bar{X}_C$, etc, etc. That is we would have to do fifteen paired tests.

ANOVA gives us a means of carrying out a preliminary test on all data at one time. This preliminary test tells us whether any pair of means among our samples is significantly different from the others, but it does not tell us which one is involved nor even how many. However, ANOVA saves a great deal of time in this respect: if our ANOVA result is not significant, it means that there is nothing to be gained by analysing the means pair by pair. On the other hand if the ANOVA result is significant, then this means that it is worthwhile checking each of the pairs for significance.

What it involves is a comparison of the variance of all of the samples.

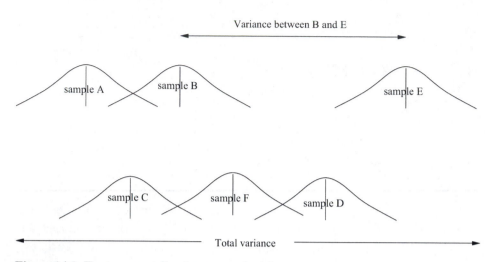

Figure 14.1 Factors contributing to total variance.

Obviously the total variance of all of the data taken together can be seen to come from two sources:

- dispersion within the individual samples – referred to as *within groups variance*
- dispersion between the means of the samples – referred to as *between groups variance.*

This can probably best be understood by means of a diagram (*see* Figure 14.1). Thus, what we do in ANOVA is to calculate a measure of dispersion within the samples, namely the variance (ANOVA only applies if the parent populations all have approximately equal variances) of a given sample, designated σ_W^2. We then calculate the variance between the sample means, designated σ_B^2.

Now it should be obvious to the reader that if the between sample variance is less than, or only equal to, the within sample variance, then the samples do not differ from one another very much. That is, if the degree of variability from treatment to treatment is no greater than the degrees of variability within any given sample, then we are not likely to conclude that one treatment is better or worse than the others.

Therefore, what we do is to consider the ratio of the two types of variances and check its magnitude for significance in the F-table (Appendix J). Since the ratio we consider is

$$F = \frac{\sigma_B^2}{\sigma_W^2}$$

then we are only interested when F is greater than one. If F is equal to one, then that means that $\sigma_B^2 = \sigma_W^2$ which would not imply significance for the reason first argued in the previous paragraph. Likewise, if F is less than one, then this would imply that there was less variability resulting from different treatments than occurred within samples of any one treatment. This would indicate that there was no significant difference between treatments and, in fact, if F was very small it would probably indicate biased sampling – matched samples, or something of that order.

Assumptions underlying ANOVA

As with every parametric statistical test, certain assumptions must be satisfied before it is even legitimate to apply ANOVA. There are three of these. They are all very important and the reader should be sure that he understands what each implies. Unless these three conditions are at least approximately met, we cannot assume that F, which we calculate by

$$F = \frac{\sigma_B^2}{\sigma_W^2}$$

is in fact distributed appropriately. If that assumption could not be made, then we would be deceiving ourselves with an appropriate table of probabilities. The three assumptions are as follows.

1 That the subjects have been assigned *randomly* to each of the treatment samples. This rules out the use of ANOVA, as described in this chapter, on matched samples or on anything other than independent samples. More sophisticated variations on the basic principles of ANOVA can equip us with parametric tools for related samples.
2 That the populations from which the samples are taken are themselves normally distributed.
3 That the variance of the populations from which the sampling was made are, or can be considered to be, equal. That is, the variances of the parent populations must be homogeneous.

Some comment should be made about each of these factors before we proceed.

Random assignment

ANOVA (as presented in this chapter) is specifically designed to meet the situation in which we are quite sure that the sampling procedure has not been biased in the direction of relating the samples to be given different treatments.

Normality of parent populations

Let the reader be reminded of just what a *population* is in statistics. If we decide to test three drugs for reducing sinus inflammation in men, we might go about it as follows.

We select 30 sufferers of sinusitis from, say, a batch of new army recruits and randomly assign them to three different treatment groups. Now the reader might suppose that all three samples have the same parent population – namely army recruits. But that is not so within the context of this experiment. We treat one sample with drug A, the next sample with drug B and the third with drug C.

Now there are three parent populations involved.

1 All of those people (not just the 10 selected) who ever will be or ever would be (hypothetically) treated with drug A – it makes no difference that drug A never existed until just prior to the experiment and that therefore no one could have been treated with it before.
2 All of those people who ever would, will or might be treated with drug B.
3 All of those people who ever would, will or might be treated with drug C.

When we specify, then, that each of these three populations must be normally distributed, even though we often cannot possibly know for sure whether they are or not (because they do not really exist yet except on paper), what we mean is this: we must have no reason, experimental or otherwise, for suspecting that the defined parent populations would deviate radically from a normal distribution.

Variance homogeneity of parent populations

Remember that if a sample variance is calculated with

$$S^2 = \frac{\Sigma_i f_i (X_i - \bar{X})^2}{N - 1}$$

instead of with

$$\sigma^2 = \frac{\Sigma_i f_i (X_i - \bar{X})^2}{N}$$

then it is an unbiased estimate of the parent population variance.

Thus, when we calculate the variance in this way for each sample, each represents an unbiased estimate of the parent population concerned. They are not likely to be identical, but we want to be as sure as possible that any difference between them is due to random factors alone and is not due to some systematic difference between the parent population variances. The parent populations can be quite different, indeed we usually hope that they are when we do ANOVA, but their variances must not be significantly different.

Developing procedures for ANOVA

Until now we have dealt with virtually no mathematics as such. We must now depart from that halcyon state of affairs and actually engage in a fair bit of numerical argument. The reader is advised to try to stick it through to the end. However, even if he cannot, all that he has to do is to follow the format laid out here and he can blindly accomplish ANOVA.

As we mentioned in the beginning of this chapter, we shall be concerned only with the simplest type of ANOVA in this book. This type of ANOVA is called 'ANOVA with one-way classification' because it is applied to observations which can be classified into sets or samples on the basis of a single property. Remember, though, these groups must be independent of one another.

For the sake of convenience, we shall consider a particular example. A clinician has tested four different methods of treating scabies in children. Five youngsters have been treated by each method. The children were then tested and the resulting data are given below.

Sample 1	Sample 2	Sample 3	Sample 4
2	3	6	2
3	4	7	3
1	2	7	5
1	4	5	5
3	2	10	5

For each sample, the sum of values is determined, the mean of each sample is obtained, as is the mean of all of the observations. As well, we calculate the sum of the squares of each observation's deviation from the grand mean. The grand mean, signified by $\bar{X}$, refers to the mean of all of the observations. This material is set out below.

	Sample 1		Sample 2		Sample 3		Sample 4		Total
	X	$(X - \bar{X})^2$	X	$(X - \bar{X})^2$	X	$(X - \bar{X})^2$	X	$(X - \bar{X})^2$	
	2	4	3	1	6	4	2	4	
	3	1	4	0	7	9	3	1	
	1	9	2	4	7	9	5	1	
	1	9	4	0	5	1	5	1	
	3	1	2	4	10	36	5	1	
ΣX	10		15		35		20		80
$\bar{X}$	2		3		7		4		
$\Sigma(X - \bar{X})^2$		24		9		59		8	100

Now, the total sum of squares, which was 100, is divided into four parts, reflecting variance *between* the samples and variance *within* the samples. We shall carefully go over the procedure involved in calculating each of these parts.

To get the between samples part, we first must eliminate the within samples part. We do this by replacing each observation by its own sample average. To get the within samples part, exactly the same procedure is followed as when the total sum of the squares was calculated. We show this in two stages.

1 We record the samples average as the value for each observation in the given sample and then compute the square of the deviation of each entry from $\tilde{X} = 4$ (*see* table below).

Sample 1		Sample2		Sample 3		Sample 4	
$\bar{X}$	$(\bar{X} - \tilde{X})^2$	$\bar{X}$	$(\bar{X} - \tilde{X})^2$	$\bar{X}$	$(\bar{X} - \tilde{X})^2$	$\bar{X}$	$(\bar{X} - \tilde{X})^2$
2	4	3	1	7	9	4	0
2	4	3	1	7	9	4	0
2	4	3	1	7	9	4	0
2	4	3	1	7	9	4	0
2	4	3	1	7	9	4	0
10	20	15	5	35	45	20	0

$$\Sigma \bar{X} = 80 \qquad \Sigma(\bar{X} - \tilde{X})^2 = 70$$

2 The next stage in our calculations is to work out the variability within the individual samples and the sum of squares of the within sample variation (*see* table opposite).

Sample 1		Sample 2		Sample 3		Sample 4	
$(X - \bar{X})$	$(X - \bar{X})^2$	$(X - \bar{X})$	$(X - \bar{X})^2$	$(X - \bar{X})$	$(X - \bar{X})^2$	$(X - \bar{X})$	$(X - \bar{X})^2$
0	0	0	0	−1	1	−2	4
+1	1	+1	1	0	0	−1	1
−1	1	−1	1	0	0	+1	1
−1	1	+1	1	−2	4	+1	1
+1	1	−1	1	+3	9	+1	1
0	4	0	4	0	14	0	8

$$\Sigma(X - \bar{X}) = 0 \qquad \Sigma(X - \bar{X})^2 = 30$$

We now come to the final stage in this incredible calculation, the stage at which we set up what is called the 'ANOVA table'. Before we proceed to show how this is done, there are one or two theoretical matters that should be touched upon.

What do the two variances mean?

First of all, how would we logically calculate the between groups variance? Well, the general formula for sample variance is

$$S^2 = \frac{\Sigma(X - \bar{X})^2}{N - 1}$$

if we want it to be an unbiased estimate of the population variance. That is, we have $(N - 1)$ degrees of freedom because we lose a degree of freedom in calculating $\bar{X}$. Now for between groups variance, we start off with k groups (*see* stage 1), but we lose one degree of freedom through calculating $\bar{X}$. Thus, when calculating between groups variance, we have $(k - 1)$ degrees of freedom. If we designate between groups variance as σ_B^2, we should get

$$\sigma_B^2 = \frac{\sum_{i=1}^{k}(\bar{X}_i - \tilde{X})^2}{k - 1}$$

Now, of what is this σ_B^2 an unbiased estimate? *It is an unbiased estimate of the population variance.* Keep that in mind.

Next let us consider the within groups variance. In order to calculate the within groups variance, we first have to calculate as many means as there are groups or samples. We agree that there are k groups (in this case $k = 4$). So if there are N observations altogether we have $(N - k)$ degrees of freedom left in calculating the within groups variance, designated σ_W^2. Therefore

$$\sigma_W^2 = \frac{\sum_{j=1}^{4} \sum_{i=1}^{5} (X_{ij} - \bar{X}_i)^2}{N - k}$$

Do not be put off by the double sigma notation, for it describes (in economical form) exactly what we did in the previous table. The inner $\sum$ means 'calculate $(X_{ij} - \bar{X}_i)^2$ for each i', there being five observations. Then we sum those values for all four samples.

$$\sum_{j=1}^{4} \sum_{i=1}^{5} (X_{ij} - \bar{X}_i)^2 = (2 - 2)^2 + (3 - 2)^2 + \ldots + (3 - 3)^2 +$$
$$(4 - 3)^2 + \ldots + (6 - 7)^2 + (7 - 7)^2 +$$
$$\ldots + (2 - 4)^2 + (3 - 4)^2 + (5 - 4)^2 +$$
$$(5 - 4)^2 + (5 - 4)^2$$
$$= 30$$

Now, of what does the within groups variance give an unbiased estimate? It is also an unbiased estimate of the population variance. Notice that we now have two unbiased estimates of σ^2, namely σ_W^2 and σ_B^2. These two estimates of the population variance are independent, because with random assignment (and that was one of the pre-conditions for carrying out ANOVA) there would be no reason to suppose that variability within groups should in any way be connected to variability between groups. Obviously, if there is no significant difference from one treatment to another, the means of the samples will be the same. In this case, σ_B^2 would equal σ_W^2 and thus

$$F = \frac{\sigma_B^2}{\sigma_W^2} = 1$$

It is when there is a difference between the sample means that although σ_B^2 and σ_W^2 are each an unbiased estimate of σ^2, the variances differ and hence produce an F ratio of interest to the investigator.

Setting up the variance table

We now know that in calculating σ_B^2 we have $(k-1)$ degrees of freedom, while in calculating σ_W^2 we have $(N-K)$ degrees of freedom. These two pieces of information, along with the computed values of σ_B^2 and σ_W^2, are all we need to set up the variance table and calculate F, bringing our ANOVA to an end. Using the data from the previous tables we now set up our variance table as follows.

Variance due to	Degrees of freedom	Sum of squares	Variance estimate
Between samples	3	70	$70/3 = 23.3$
Within samples	16	30	$30/16 = 1.9$

$$F = \frac{23.3}{1.9} = 12.3$$

Using the F-table in Appendix J, degrees of freedom 3 and 16, we check at the 0.01 significance level and we find that a value equal or in excess of 5.29 would be significant. Since our computed F-value was 12.3, we conclude that this result is significant. That means that we conclude that at least one of our four treatments was significantly different from the rest: knowing that, we would probably find it worthwhile to examine them pair by pair until we isolate the ones responsible.

Discussion of steps in ANOVA

Now that the reader has some intuitive grasp of what ANOVA is all about and has actually followed through the calculations associated with ANOVA, he should be prepared to consider in greater depth the steps that we have taken. Some confusion may be caused by the use of the double sigma notation, so we shall proceed to eliminate that problem first.

Consider the array of numbers that follows:

1	0	4	1	7	2	3
5	1	9	0	4	6	8
2	2	1	5	7	2	5

Let i designate the rows and j represent the columns so that for $j = 4$

$$\sum_{i=1}^{3} x_i = 1 + 0 + 5 = 6$$

because when j is fixed at 4 we are saying 'consider the fourth column'. That is, the rows are numbered from 1 to 3 starting at the top and the columns are numbered from 1 to 7 starting at the left.

Therefore, x_{ij} refers to the element in the ith row and the jth column, so that $x_{25} = 4$ (the number in the second row, fifth column). This simple notation can be used to describe rather involved sums. For example,

$$\sum_{j=1}^{4} \sum_{i=1}^{3} x_{ij} \text{ means}[(1 + 5 + 2) + (0 + 1 + 2)$$
$$+ (4 + 9 + 1) + (1 + 0 + 5)]$$

So

$$\sum_{j=1}^{4} \sum_{i=1}^{3} x_{ij} = 31$$

Now the reader will remember that we considered the contributions made to the total dispersion of scores by the dispersion within the sample and the dispersion between the means of the samples. We shall now go over this ground again more systematically. If the grand mean is $\tilde{X}$, then the deviation of any given score from it is given by $(X_{ij} - \tilde{X})$. Now where X_j is the mean of any given sample, this deviation can be written as

$$X_{ij} - \tilde{X} = (X_{ij} - \bar{X}_j) + (\bar{X}_j - \tilde{X})$$

Let us square both sides of this equation

$$(X_{ij} - \tilde{X})^2 = (X_{ij} - \bar{X}_j)^2 + (\bar{X}_j - \tilde{X})^2 + 2(X_{ij} - \bar{X}_j)(\bar{X}_j - \tilde{X})$$

Sum both sides of the equation on both i and j. Therefore where there are n in each sample and k samples

$$\sum_{j=1}^{k} \sum_{i=1}^{n} (X_{ij} - \tilde{X})^2 = \sum_{j=1}^{k} \sum_{i=1}^{n} (X_{ij} - \bar{X}_j)^2 + \sum_{j=1}^{k} \sum_{i=1}^{n} (\bar{X}_j - \tilde{X})^2$$

the reader may wonder what happened to the third term on the right hand side, namely

$$\sum_{j=1}^{k}\sum_{i=1}^{n}(X_{ij} - \bar{X}_j)(\bar{X}_j - \tilde{X})$$

The reason that term vanishes is because $\sum_{i=1}^{n}(X_{ij} - -\bar{X}_j) = 0$. Try it out on

4	3	5	6
5	2	4	7
6	1	3	8

$$\bar{X}_1 = 5; \bar{X}_2 = 2; \bar{X}_3 = 4; \bar{X}_4 = 7; \tilde{X} = 4.5.$$

So

$$\sum_{j=1}^{4}\sum_{i=1}^{3}(X_{ij} - \bar{X}_j) = [(4 - 5) + (5 - 5) + (6 - 5)]+$$
$$[(3 - 2) + (2 - 2) + (1 - 2)]+$$
$$[(5 - 4) + (4 - 4) + (3 - 4)]+$$
$$[(6 - 7) + (7 - 7) + (8 - 7)]$$
$$= 0 + 0 + 0 + 0$$
$$= 0$$

Thus we have

$$\sum_{j=1}^{k}\sum_{i=1}^{n}(X_{ij} - \tilde{X})^2 = \sum_{j=1}^{k}\sum_{i=1}^{n}(X_{ij} - \bar{X}_j)^2 + \sum_{j=1}^{k}\sum_{i=1}^{n}(\bar{X}_j - \tilde{X})^2$$

Let us examine these two components carefully. $(X_{ij} - \tilde{X})^2$ is the square of the deviation of each score, from the grand mean. Thus we call $\Sigma\Sigma(X_{ij} - \tilde{X})^2$ the Total Sum of Squares or TSS. $(X_{ij} - \bar{X}_j)^2$ is the square of the deviation of each score, from its sample mean. Thus we call $\Sigma\Sigma(X_{ij} - \bar{X}_j)^2$ the Within Samples Sum of Squares or WSS. $(\bar{X}_j - \tilde{X})^2$ is the square of the deviation of each sample mean, from the grand mean. Thus we call $\Sigma\Sigma(\bar{X}_j - \tilde{X})^2$ the Between Samples Sum of Squares or BSS. Therefore, we can say that

$TSS = WSS + BSS$. This discovery enables us to partition the variance according to the components contributed by within sample variance and between samples variance respectively. This is because, as we have already seen

$$\sigma^2 = \frac{\sum_{j=1}^{k} \sum_{i=1}^{n} (X_{ij} - \tilde{X})^2}{N - 1}$$

$$= \frac{TSS}{N - 1}$$

$$\sigma_W^2 = \frac{\sum_{j=1}^{k} \sum_{i=1}^{n} (X_{ij} - \bar{X}_j)^2}{N - k}$$

$$= \frac{WSS}{N - 1}$$

$$\sigma_B^2 = \frac{\sum_{j=1}^{k} \sum_{i=1}^{n} (\bar{X}_j - \tilde{X})^2}{k - 1}$$

$$= \frac{BSS}{N - 1}$$

It is figures derived from these calculations, then, which allow us to generate a general variance table, as shown below.

Variance due to	Degrees of freedom	Sum of squares (SS)	Variance estimate
Between samples	$k - 1$	BSS	σ_B^2
Within samples	$N - k$	WSS	σ_W^2
Total	$N - 1$	TSS	$F = \dfrac{\sigma_B^2}{\sigma_W^2}$

An ANOVA problem

We shall work another problem right through to be sure that the reader understands what he is doing.

A psychologist is conducting an experiment on fear reduction as measured by a test giving numerical results. He exposes three unrelated samples of subjects (20 in each sample) to three different treatments and then tests them. His results were as shown in the table opposite.

	Treatment A	Treatment B	Treatment C
	52	28	15
	48	35	14
	43	34	23
	50	32	21
	43	34	14
	44	27	20
	46	31	21
	46	27	16
	43	29	20
	49	25	14
	38	43	23
	42	34	25
	42	33	18
	35	42	26
	33	41	18
	38	37	26
	39	37	20
	34	40	19
	33	36	22
	34	35	17
Total	832	680	392

When we have a calculation as massive as this to carry out, it would take ages if we merely used the formulae for BSS and WSS as developed in the last section. However, it is heartening to note that the formulae for BSS and WSS have been proven to be equivalent to a simpler form, which we ordinarily rely on in calculations.

Thus

$$WSS = \sum\sum(X_{ij} - \bar{X}_j)^2$$

$$= \sum_{j=1}^{k}\sum_{i=1}^{n}(X_{ij}^2) - \frac{1}{n}\sum_{j=1}^{k}\left(\sum_{i=1}^{n}X_{ij}\right)^2$$

and

$$BSS = \sum\sum(\bar{X}_j - \tilde{X})^2$$

$$= \frac{1}{n}\sum_{j=1}^{k}\left(\sum_{i=1}^{n}X_{ij}\right)^2 - \frac{1}{N}\left(\sum_{j=1}^{k}\sum_{i=1}^{n}X_{ij}\right)^2$$

and

$$TSS = \sum\sum(X_{ij} - \tilde{X})^2$$

$$= \sum_{j=1}^{k}\sum_{i=1}^{n}(X_{ij}^2) - \frac{1}{N}\left(\sum_{j=1}^{k}\sum_{i=1}^{n}X_{ij}\right)^2$$

Now using our data from the table we can calculate

$$WSS = 66872 - 65414.4 = 1457.6$$

$$BSS = 65414.4 - 60420.3 = 4994.1$$

$$TSS = 66872 - \frac{(1904)^2}{60} = 6451.7$$

Needless to say, calculations like this are rarely worked out by paper and pencil, but almost invariably involve the use of a calculator or, better still, a computer! Our variance table now looks as follows.

Variance due to	Degrees of freedom	Sum of squares	Variance estimate
Between samples	$3 - 1 = 2$	4994.1	2497.1
Within samples	$60 - 3 = 57$	1457.6	25.6
Total	$60 - 1 = 59$	6451.7	109.4

$$F = \frac{2497.1}{25.6} = 97.5$$

On looking in the F-table at the 0.05 level with 2 and 57 degrees of freedom, an F-value equal to or in excess of 3.2 is required for significance. Since our computed value of F is much larger than that, we are certainly justified in coming to the conclusion that one of the treatments A, B or C was markedly different in its effects from the other two.

But why use ANOVA?

Although we have now explained what ANOVA is, the reader might well be forgiven for asking why he should ever use it when he has, say, the Student t-test. To use ANOVA in a situation in which the t-test would have served as well would be very much in the order of hunting butterflies with a machine gun!

ANOVA allows us to consider the problem of determining whether among a set of more than two samples, one or more of the population means differs markedly from the others. The t-test, of course, only allows us to do this with two means, but the ANOVA could still be sidestepped by considering every possible pair of the means involved. This involves extra work, of course, but anyone who is frightened of the sophistication of ANOVA might gladly put forth the necessary exertions.

Looked at more closely, though, one can see that such a use of the t-test could easily lead to a false conclusion. A simple example makes the point rather tellingly.

Suppose we have seven samples from populations the means of which are all equal. Use of combinatorial algebra shows us (by calculating the number of different pairs from seven objects) that we would have to carry out 21 t-tests. Obviously, for each of these, the probability of coming to the right conclusion that no significant difference exists must be 0.95 if $\alpha = 0.05$. Thus, the probability that we would reach the right conclusion on all 21 pairs would be $(0.95)^{21} = 0.34$. In that case, the probability of obtaining at least one incorrect solution is given by $1 - 0.34 = 0.66$. Therefore, 66 percent of the time we would be coming to the wrong conclusion by committing a Type 1 error. Such a consideration means that the proposed procedure would be clearly unacceptable, especially when one realises that for larger numbers of samples the chances of making a Type 1 error would be even greater.

It is for this reason that ANOVA was developed, for it allows us to consider all of the sample means simultaneously.

Chapter 15

A brief introduction to designing a research project

Formulating your research problem

A good research problem best arises naturally in the context of practice, rather than being contrived for the sake of an impressive data display. At first, the idea is very general. Don't artificially restrict your enquiries at the outset through what you perceive as being 'analytical limitations'. Analytical limitations can be of two types.

1 You are apprehensive about your own grasp of statistics and hesitate, therefore, to embark on a project which you suspect will involve sophisticated techniques.
2 You ask a question for which mathematics has not yet devised a satisfactory analytical approach.

Let neither of these deter you. With respect to (1), you just need to have the faintest idea of what you want, and any number of statistics handbooks are available to tell you exactly what to do. As far as (2) is concerned, go ahead and formulate the question. If the limitation you perceive is real, none of the handbooks will help you. You then go to a statistics lecturer (but retain your copyright of the question – just in case!). If they cannot help you, the question will be referred to a mathematician dealing with that field. If you really have found a gap, you will be informed and thus have the basis for an interesting communication to a statistical research journal. It is not often that simply the question leads to a publication, but it has happened!

Think right now of some very general research questions that can arise in your field of healthcare, e.g. effect of training sessions on interpersonal skills in engendering patient confidence in the practitioner; does osteopathy reduce the incidence of pre-eclampsia in pregnancy, etc.? There are no limits! Notice that the phrasing of the initial general question totally ignores such strategic considerations as how to measure the variables. Get your priorities right; let your genuine professional curiosity govern the questions you ask and only refine them later in the light of restrictions imposed by data collection problems, ethics, etc. This 'refining' process is best carried out in consultation with more experienced colleagues, a statistician or two, the Ethics Committee, etc. But the important thing to remember is that the first step in research design is to *ask a question.*

Now, even before refining the question, consider your *resources.* Do you have access to the data? If you need clinical data, do you (or your colleagues) see enough patients to obtain it? If a 'before' and 'after' situation is envisaged, does your situation permit collection of data at frequent enough intervals?

After you have satisfied yourself with respect to these details, you need to seek professional advice to ascertain whether the question has already been asked and answered. Just because the idea is original to you does not necessarily mean that it is original to the profession. Often, all the professional advice you need in this regard can be provided by a good medical librarian. More often, you will have to check with your research director first, who, in collaboration with the librarian, can see whether the matter has already been resolved. This step is called 'surveying the literature'.

At this point, if you are honestly sure that the ground has not already been trodden, you set down and elaborate your *research protocol.* This includes asking the question as unambiguously as possible and stating in precise detail how you propose to answer it. It is possibly the most difficult part of the whole process and the restrictions will come at you thick and fast. For instance, is it ethical? You would think that such a question would be easy. Not so. Suppose you had reason to believe that a particular 5-minute manipulation of a pregnant patient's feet significantly reduced the incidence of discomfort caused by oedema. OK, how would you find out? I suppose you could do it to every second patient you saw from the first trimester through to delivery and then analyse the difference between those to whom it was done and those to whom it wasn't.

But, hold on! Suppose it does work? Then, you have knowingly deprived certain patients of benefits by withholding a technique that certainly would not have harmed them, even if it had not worked. Was that ethical? Well, you would have to be a Solomon or a Daniel come to judgement to determine such things. Fortunately, you rarely have to do so unaided. The people who run the facility in which you are taking the data have to make those decisions, so you consult them when you have worked out your protocol. In most cases they, in turn, will be able to consult an Ethics Committee. In reviewing your proposal, the people who run the facility will not only consider the ethics involved, although that is the most crucial consideration; they will also advise as to whether or not the proposal is financially feasible; whether it can be carried out in the time allocated, etc. Your research protocol needs to be written up so well (including a literature review) that anyone else with your training could carry out the experiment precisely as you would. The next section will tell you how to do this.

Thus, to summarise:

1 Ask a general question.
2 Look into your resources for answering it.
3 Do a literature survey.
4 Refine your research protocol in consultation with your supervisors.
5 Write up the research proposal.

Writing up the proposal

You must always begin with the statement of 'Aims and Objectives'. Are you clear as to the difference? 'Aims and Objectives' is a phrase used by all sorts of people and has a professional 'ring' to it, but many who use it think it simply is a rather redundant way of saying 'purpose'. No, 'aims' and 'objectives' are two separate issues. The 'aims' reflect the general intention of the project (e.g. 'to ascertain if . . .') while the 'objectives' state the steps that you will take to achieve the 'aims'. There is absolutely no room for confusion here. First, be completely clear in your own mind as to what your aims are and what objectives have to be satisfied to achieve them. Then, write them unambiguously.

Here is an example.

Aims

1 To ascertain whether osteopathic treatment of sprains affects the recovery of previously existing muscle tone in the sprained area.
2 To determine whether patient awareness of improvement correlates with the recovery of muscle tone.

Objectives

1 To review the literature.
2 To select a sample of unilateral sprains so that comparisons can be made from time to time with the uninjured side in the same patient.
3 To analyse the data obtained and use it to satisfy the aims.
4 To enunciate conclusions in terms of these findings.

Revising, doing, revising

Notice that in the 'objectives' we do not go into details of methodology. How do we make the comparisons mentioned in item 2? How are we going to analyse the data as mentioned in item 3? All of that is detailed in 'Methods'. Also, it needs to be borne in mind that the statement of Aims and Objectives may have to be modified, possibly even changed altogether, as a result of further 'progress' with the project. For instance, suppose that you have six weeks in which to collect your data (that is something that you establish when 'looking into resources') and you then find out that permission you need for a particular objective (or part thereof) can only be obtained from a committee which is not due to convene for another two months. Obviously, in that event, the objectives have to be changed. If they have to be altered drastically because of unexpected events, you then have to reconsider the aims. The important thing is not to feel a 'loyalty' to your protocol so strongly as to compromise your integrity. A shoddy experiment is not worth doing, and one with spurious data even less so. A well-done project, even if inferior in scope, is always of value.

For people who have never done research, it is this sense of 'changing plans and altering blueprints' while the building is in progress, that causes the most anxiety. The history of science is very rarely taught in most routine science courses, with the result that people come to research with the idea that 'proper' research is carried out as originally conceived and that the necessity to keep changing the scope and even the thrust of a project necessarily suggest an inadequate investigator. That this is not true can readily be appreciated by reading even a layman's account of any great scientific project. Even great monuments to scientific thought; theories of evolution and of relativity, the laws of thermodynamics, Mendelian trait segregation, Freudian psychoanalysis, etc., all emerged from patched-up protocols.

Let us assume that you are finally doing the experiment, generating the data that will be analysed. This requires that your Method, although perhaps re-stated several times, has been explicitly written out. At that point, and before actually generating your data (by whatever means), you must work out what statistical analysis you intend to use. Many research projects have foundered not through lack of data, but through the wrong kind of data. You will be much more aware of the sort of thing to which reference is being made after you have studied the sections on 'sampling' and 'testing'. Suffice to say, you should discuss this aspect of it with a statistician or with your research project director prior to collecting the data. The tests that you want to use, or were thinking of using, may require a particular form of data, a novel method of asking questions, etc.

Answers to study exercises

Study exercises 1

1 (a) 8.4.
  (b) The median is between 9.2 and 11.3, split the difference, 10.25.
  (c) The mean deviation is 1.41.
  (d) The standard deviation is 3.84.

2 Set up the data as follows, once you have calculated the mean:

Class boundary	x (midpoint)	f	$\lvert x - m \rvert$	$f\lvert x - m \rvert$	$(x - m)^2$	$f(x - m)^2$
10–30	20	5				
30–50	40	8				
50–70	60	12				
70–90	80	18				
90–110	100	3				
110–130	120	2				

Stop at this point to calculate the group mean. The total number, n, is $\Sigma f = 48$.

(a)
$$\frac{\Sigma fx}{n} = \frac{3120}{48} = 65$$

(b) There are 48 scores, you want the score above (and below) which 24 fall. Start adding up the frequencies: $5 + 8 + 12 = 25$, so the median is in the class 50–70. In that class 12 scores fall, you want 11 more.

$$\frac{11}{12} \times 20 = frac553 = 18.33$$

So the median is $50 + 18.33 = 68.33$.

(c) The modal class is the interval with the highest frequency: 70–90. Now you can fill in the columns: $\lvert x - m \rvert$, $f\lvert x - m \rvert$, $(x - m)^2$, $f(x - m)^2$.

Class boundary	x (midpoint)	f	$\|x - m\|$	$f\|x - m\|$	$(x - m)^2$	$f(x - m)^2$
10–30	20	5	45	225	50625	253125
30–50	40	8	25	200	40000	320000
50–70	60	12	5	60	3600	43200
70–90	80	18	15	270	72900	1312200
90–110	100	3	35	105	11025	33075
110–130	120	2	55	110	12100	24200

(d) The mean deviation is simply

$$\frac{970}{48} = 20.208 = 20.21$$

(e) The variance would be $\frac{1985800}{47} = 42251.063$. Take its square root to get the standard deviation

$$sd = \sqrt{42251.063} = 205.55$$

3   This problem is done in exactly the same way.

Study exercises 2

1   $\frac{4}{13}$

2   $\frac{5}{18}$

3   $\frac{13}{18}$

4   $\frac{1}{462}$

5   $\frac{11}{425}$

6   (a) 0.0005
    (b) 0.0590
    (c) $1 - (0.0590 + 0.0005) = 1 - 0.0595 = 0.9405$

7   $\frac{7}{12}$

8   $\frac{91}{648}$

9   (a) $\frac{1}{216}$

    (b) $\frac{1}{36}$

    (c) $\frac{5}{72}$

(d) $\frac{5}{12}$

(e) $\frac{5}{9}$

10 360

11 120

12 (a) 210
    (b) 371

13 (a) 35
    (b) 15

14 5760

15 8400

16 (a) $\frac{280}{2187}$

    (b) $\frac{232}{243}$

Study exercises 3

1 3.50

2 $\frac{7}{10}$

3 15.1263, 32.4135, 27.7830, 11.9070, 2.5515, 0.2187

Study exercises 4

1 (a) 0.0606
   (b) You work it out!

Study exercises 6

1 $P = 0.0646$ for a two-tailed test, so not significant.

2 7

Study exercises 7

1 (a) Straight
   (b) Not straight

(c) Not straight

(d) Straight – parallel with y-axis

(e) Straight

2   (a) SR

(b) KL

(c) QP

(d) AB

(e) The line is vertical.

3   (a) $m = \frac{1}{4}$

(b) $m = \frac{21}{2}$

(c) $m = 0$. The line is horizontal.

(d) $m = 0$. The line is horizontal.

(e) m is undefined. If there is no horizontal displacement, how can the slope be defined?

4   (a) $y = \frac{2}{4}x - \frac{5}{4}$; $m = \frac{1}{2}$, $b = -\frac{5}{4}$

(b) $t = -\frac{3}{5}s + 9$; $m = -\frac{3}{5}$, $b = 9$

(c) $l = \frac{5}{6}k - 2$; $m = \frac{5}{6}$, $b = -2$

5   $3y - x = -11$

6   $3y = 2x + 6$

Study exercises 8

1   (a) -0.92

(b) 2.66

(c) 0.85

Appendix A

Areas under the normal probability curve (*Z*-table)

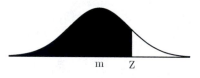

Figure A.1 Values denote the area under the standardised normal curve to the left of the given *Z*-value.

Z	0.00	0.01	0.02	0.03	0.04	0.05	0.06	0.07	0.08	0.09
0.0	0.5000	0.5040	0.5080	0.5120	0.5160	0.5199	0.5239	0.5279	0.5319	0.5359
0.1	0.5398	0.5438	0.5478	0.5517	0.5557	0.5596	0.5636	0.5675	0.5714	0.5753
0.2	0.5793	0.5832	0.5871	0.5910	0.5948	0.5987	0.6026	0.6064	0.6103	0.6141
0.3	0.6179	0.6217	0.6255	0.6293	0.6331	0.6368	0.6406	0.6443	0.6480	0.6517
0.4	0.6554	0.6591	0.6628	0.6664	0.6700	0.6736	0.6772	0.6808	0.6844	0.6879
0.5	0.6915	0.6950	0.6985	0.7019	0.7054	0.7088	0.7123	0.7157	0.7190	0.7224
0.6	0.7257	0.7291	0.7324	0.7357	0.7389	0.7422	0.7454	0.7486	0.7517	0.7549
0.7	0.7580	0.7611	0.7642	0.7673	0.7703	0.7734	0.7764	0.7794	0.7823	0.7852
0.8	0.7881	0.7910	0.7939	0.7967	0.7995	0.8023	0.8051	0.8078	0.8106	0.8133
0.9	0.8159	0.8186	0.8212	0.8238	0.8264	0.8289	0.8315	0.8340	0.8365	0.8389
1.0	0.8413	0.8438	0.8461	0.8485	0.8508	0.8531	0.8554	0.8577	0.8599	0.8621
1.1	0.8643	0.8665	0.8686	0.8708	0.8729	0.8749	0.8770	0.8790	0.8810	0.8830
1.2	0.8849	0.8869	0.8888	0.8907	0.8925	0.8944	0.8962	0.8980	0.8997	0.9015
1.3	0.9032	0.9049	0.9066	0.9082	0.9099	0.9115	0.9131	0.9147	0.9162	0.9177
1.4	0.9192	0.9207	0.9222	0.9236	0.9251	0.9265	0.9279	0.9292	0.9306	0.9319
1.5	0.9332	0.9345	0.9357	0.9370	0.9382	0.9394	0.9406	0.9418	0.9429	0.9441
1.6	0.9452	0.9463	0.9474	0.9484	0.9495	0.9505	0.9515	0.9525	0.9535	0.9545
1.7	0.9554	0.9564	0.9573	0.9582	0.9591	0.9599	0.9608	0.9616	0.9625	0.9633
1.8	0.9641	0.9649	0.9656	0.9664	0.9671	0.9678	0.9686	0.9693	0.9699	0.9706
1.9	0.9713	0.9719	0.9726	0.9732	0.9738	0.9744	0.9750	0.9756	0.9761	0.9767
2.0	0.9772	0.9778	0.9783	0.9788	0.9793	0.9798	0.9803	0.9808	0.9812	0.9817
2.1	0.9821	0.9826	0.9830	0.9834	0.9838	0.9842	0.9846	0.9850	0.9854	0.9857
2.2	0.9861	0.9864	0.9868	0.9871	0.9875	0.9878	0.9881	0.9884	0.9887	0.9890
2.3	0.9893	0.9896	0.9898	0.9901	0.9904	0.9906	0.9909	0.9911	0.9913	0.9916
2.4	0.9918	0.9920	0.9922	0.9925	0.9927	0.9929	0.9931	0.9932	0.9934	0.9936
2.5	0.9938	0.9940	0.9941	0.9943	0.9945	0.9946	0.9948	0.9949	0.9951	0.9952
2.6	0.9953	0.9955	0.9956	0.9957	0.9959	0.9960	0.9961	0.9962	0.9963	0.9964
2.7	0.9965	0.9966	0.9967	0.9968	0.9969	0.9970	0.9971	0.9972	0.9973	0.9974

Z	0.00	0.01	0.02	0.03	0.04	0.05	0.06	0.07	0.08	0.09
2.8	0.9974	0.9975	0.9976	0.9977	0.9977	0.9978	0.9979	0.9979	0.9980	0.9981
2.9	0.9981	0.9982	0.9982	0.9983	0.9984	0.9984	0.9985	0.9985	0.9986	0.9986
3.0	0.9987	0.9987	0.9987	0.9988	0.9988	0.9989	0.9989	0.9989	0.9990	0.9990
3.1	0.9990	0.9991	0.9991	0.9991	0.9992	0.9992	0.9992	0.9992	0.9993	0.9993
3.2	0.9993	0.9993	0.9994	0.9994	0.9994	0.9994	0.9994	0.9995	0.9995	0.9995
3.3	0.9995	0.9995	0.9995	0.9996	0.9996	0.9996	0.9996	0.9996	0.9996	0.9997
3.4	0.9997	0.9997	0.9997	0.9997	0.9997	0.9997	0.9997	0.9997	0.9997	0.9998
3.5	0.9998	0.9998	0.9998	0.9998	0.9998	0.9998	0.9998	0.9998	0.9998	0.9998
3.6	0.9998	0.9998	0.9999	0.9999	0.9999	0.9999	0.9999	0.9999	0.9999	0.9999
3.7	0.9999	0.9999	0.9999	0.9999	0.9999	0.9999	0.9999	0.9999	0.9999	0.9999
3.8	0.9999	0.9999	0.9999	0.9999	0.9999	0.9999	0.9999	0.9999	0.9999	0.9999
3.9	1.0000	1.0000	1.0000	1.0000	1.0000	1.0000	1.0000	1.0000	1.0000	1.0000

Appendix B

Distribution of *t*

DF	0.5	0.1	0.05	0.02	0.01	0.002
1	1.000	6.314	12.706	31.821	63.657	318.31
2	0.816	2.920	4.303	6.965	9.925	22.327
3	0.765	2.353	3.182	4.541	5.841	10.215
4	0.741	2.132	2.776	3.747	4.604	7.173
5	0.727	2.015	2.571	3.365	4.032	5.893
6	0.718	1.943	2.447	3.143	3.707	5.208
7	0.711	1.895	2.365	2.998	3.499	4.785
8	0.706	1.860	2.306	2.896	3.355	4.501
9	0.703	1.833	2.262	2.821	3.250	4.297
10	0.700	1.812	2.228	2.764	3.169	4.144
11	0.697	1.796	2.201	2.718	3.106	4.025
12	0.695	1.782	2.179	2.681	3.055	3.930
13	0.694	1.771	2.160	2.650	3.012	3.852
14	0.692	1.761	2.145	2.624	2.977	3.787
15	0.691	1.753	2.131	2.602	2.947	3.733
16	0.690	1.746	2.120	2.583	2.921	3.686
17	0.689	1.740	2.110	2.567	2.898	3.646
18	0.688	1.734	2.101	2.552	2.878	3.610
19	0.688	1.729	2.093	2.539	2.861	3.579
20	0.687	1.725	2.086	2.528	2.845	3.552
21	0.686	1.721	2.080	2.518	2.831	3.527
22	0.686	1.717	2.074	2.508	2.819	3.505
23	0.685	1.714	2.069	2.500	2.807	3.485
24	0.685	1.711	2.064	2.492	2.797	3.467
25	0.684	1.708	2.060	2.485	2.787	3.450
26	0.684	1.706	2.056	2.479	2.779	3.435
27	0.684	1.703	2.052	2.473	2.771	3.421
28	0.683	1.701	2.048	2.467	2.763	3.408
29	0.683	1.699	2.045	2.462	2.756	3.396
30	0.683	1.697	2.042	2.457	2.750	3.385
35	0.682	1.690	2.030	2.438	2.724	3.340
40	0.681	1.684	2.021	2.423	2.704	3.307
45	0.680	1.679	2.014	2.412	2.690	3.281
50	0.679	1.676	2.009	2.403	2.678	3.261
55	0.679	1.673	2.004	2.396	2.668	3.245
60	0.679	1.671	2.000	2.390	2.660	3.232
∞	0.674	1.645	1.960	2.326	2.576	3.090

Appendix C

Wilcoxon distribution (with no pairing)

The numbers given in this table are the number of cases for which the sum of the ranks of the sample of size n_1 is less than or equal to W_1. The columns denote values of U, where $U = W_1 - \frac{1}{2}n_1(n_1 + 1)$.

n_1	n_2	C_{n_1,n_2}	0	1	2	3	4	5	6	7	8	9	10
3	3	20	1	2	4	7	10	13	16	18	19	20	
3	4	35	1	2	4	7	11	15	20	24	28	31	33
4	4	70	1	2	4	7	12	17	24	31	39	46	53
3	5	56	1	2	4	7	11	16	22	28	34	40	45
4	5	126	1	2	4	7	12	18	26	35	46	57	69
5	5	252	1	2	4	7	12	19	28	39	53	69	87
3	6	84	1	2	4	7	11	16	23	30	38	46	54
4	6	210	1	2	4	7	12	18	27	37	50	64	80
5	6	462	1	2	4	7	12	19	29	41	57	76	99
6	6	924	1	2	4	7	12	19	30	43	61	83	111
3	7	120	1	2	4	7	11	16	23	31	40	50	60
4	7	330	1	2	4	7	12	18	27	38	52	68	87
5	7	792	1	2	4	7	12	19	29	42	59	80	106
6	7	1716	1	2	4	7	12	19	30	44	63	87	118
7	7	3432	1	2	4	7	12	19	30	45	65	91	125
3	8	165	1	2	4	7	11	16	23	31	41	52	64
4	8	495	1	2	4	7	12	18	27	38	53	70	91
5	8	1287	1	2	4	7	12	19	29	42	60	82	110
6	8	3003	1	2	4	7	12	19	30	44	64	89	122
7	8	6435	1	2	4	7	12	19	30	45	66	93	129
8	8	12870	1	2	4	7	12	19	30	45	67	95	133

n_1	n_2	C_{n_1,n_2}	11	12	13	14	15	16	17	18	19	20
3	3	20										
3	4	35	34	35								
4	4	70	58	63	66	68	69	70				
3	5	56	49	52	54	55	56					
4	5	126	80	91	100	108	114	119	122	124	125	126
5	5	252	106	126	146	165	183	199	213	224	233	240
3	6	84	61	68	73	77	80	82	83	84		
4	6	210	96	114	130	146	160	173	183	192	198	203
5	6	462	124	153	183	215	247	279	309	338	363	386
6	6	924	143	182	224	272	323	378	433	491	546	601
3	7	120	70	80	89	97	104	109	113	116	118	119
4	7	330	107	130	153	177	200	223	243	262	278	292
5	7	792	136	171	210	253	299	347	396	445	493	539
6	7	1716	155	201	253	314	382	458	539	627	717	811
7	7	3432	167	220	283	358	445	545	657	782	918	1064
3	8	165	76	89	101	113	124	134	142	149	154	158
4	8	495	114	141	169	200	231	264	295	326	354	381
5	8	1287	143	183	228	280	337	400	466	536	607	680
6	8	3003	162	213	272	343	424	518	621	737	860	994
7	8	6435	174	232	302	388	489	609	746	904	1080	1277
8	8	12870	181	244	321	418	534	675	839	1033	1254	1509

Appendix D

Wilcoxon distribution (with pairing) where $W_1 \leq n$

The numbers given in this table are the number of cases for which the sum of the ranks is less than or equal to W_1.

W_1		W_1		W_1		W_1	
0	1						
1	2	6	14	11	55	16	169
2	3	7	19	12	70	17	207
3	5	8	25	13	88	18	253
4	7	9	33	14	110	19	307
5	10	10	43	15	137	20	371

Appendix E

Wilcoxon distribution (with pairing) where $W_1 > n$

$W_1 - n$	$n = 3$	4	5	6	7	8	9	10	11
1	6	9	13	18	24	32	42	54	69
2	7	11	16	22	30	40	52	67	85
3	8	13	19	27	37	49	64	82	104
4		14	22	32	44	59	77	99	126
5		15	325	37	52	70	92	119	151
6		16	27	42	60	82	109	141	179
7			29	46	68	95	127	165	211
8			30	50	76	108	146	192	246
9			31	54	84	121	167	221	285
10			32	57	91	135	188	252	328
11				59	98	148	210	285	374
12				61	104	161	253	320	423
13				62	109	174	256	356	476
14				63	114	186	279	394	532
15				64	118	197	302	433	591
16					121	207	324	472	653
17					123	216	345	512	717
18					125	224	366	552	783
19					126	231	385	591	851
20					127	237	403	630	920
21					128	242	420	668	989
22						246	435	704	1059
23						249	448	739	1128
24						251	460	772	1197
25						253	470	803	1265
26						254	479	832	1331
27						255	487	859	1395
28						256	493	883	1457
29							498	905	1516
30							502	925	1572

$W_1 - n$	$n = 12$	13	14	15	16	17	18	19	20
1	87	109	136	168	206	252	306	370	446
2	107	134	166	204	250	304	368	444	533
3	131	163	201	247	301	365	441	530	634
4	158	196	242	296	360	436	525	629	751
5	189	235	289	353	429	518	622	744	886
6	225	279	343	419	508	612	734	876	1041
7	265	329	405	494	598	720	862	1027	1219
8	310	386	475	579	701	843	1008	1200	1422
9	361	450	554	676	818	983	1175	1397	1653
10	417	521	643	785	950	1142	1364	1620	1916
11	478	600	742	907	1099	1321	1577	1873	2213
12	545	687	852	1044	1266	1522	1818	2158	2548
13	617	782	974	1196	1452	1748	2088	2478	2926
14	695	886	1108	1364	1660	2000	2390	2838	3350
15	779	999	1254	1550	1890	2280	2728	3240	3825
16	868	1120	1414	1753	2143	2591	3103	3688	4356
17	962	1251	1587	1975	2422	2934	3519	4187	4947
18	1062	1391	1774	2218	2728	3312	3980	4740	5604
19	1166	1539	1976	2481	3062	3728	4487	5351	6333
20	1274	1697	2192	2766	3427	4183	5045	6026	7139
21	1387	1863	2433	3074	3823	4680	5658	6769	8028
22	1502	2037	2669	3404	4251	5222	6328	7584	9008
23	1620	2219	2929	3757	4714	5810	7059	8478	10084
24	1741	2408	3203	4135	5212	6447	7856	9455	11264
25	1863	2603	3492	4536	5746	7136	8721	10520	12557
26	1986	2805	3794	4961	6318	7878	9658	11681	13968
27	2110	3012	4109	5411	6928	8675	10673	12941	15506
28	2233	3223	4437	5884	7576	9531	11766	14306	17180
29	2355	3438	4776	6380	8265	10445	12942	15783	18997
30	2476	3656	5126	6901	8993	11420	14206	17377	20966

Appendix F

Random numbers

	(1)	(2)	(3)	(4)	(5)	(6)	(7)	(8)
1	80373	45217	57966	15643	95146	84961	30539	03255
2	64237	60896	46485	29648	19237	13166	19841	00248
3	34713	68301	81411	55819	96722	66400	57437	01460
4	89249	85161	27526	31331	18536	27386	81128	98910
5	72603	55447	30905	84101	40408	61445	87357	04645
6	38693	33842	50645	57930	63360	70487	74531	98073
7	38788	55942	53892	51863	38694	27681	69675	27943
8	12842	97201	59274	31379	40940	56754	46641	13543
9	12201	77546	97645	68962	55343	01354	89959	94037
10	35196	40605	68319	98556	11092	42850	12981	66232
11	15144	83226	34447	53838	10907	04122	98133	23750
12	17676	73759	71481	58616	30514	18122	88511	59067
13	12020	02508	28029	67364	03862	17989	77753	55410
14	58594	46072	70318	69686	05275	99652	52270	36771
15	82878	86718	06962	93785	90840	05095	33887	24868
16	95207	05368	83484	25721	39842	88348	01140	51863
17	90856	29170	35579	11071	47159	13332	82833	22105
18	75756	53152	91791	97383	52804	60413	34155	35682
19	47131	57469	45819	54324	78916	96059	95544	74123
20	17779	95381	16196	57622	83729	17337	25837	90937
21	46507	61416	02008	10018	91100	84842	32123	66856
22	54346	40266	80592	07150	00679	31099	59184	64163
23	88568	21355	34839	67484	33766	30383	57960	51546
24	42116	74156	25520	25845	07845	51357	33135	70704
25	29125	35143	80722	20225	36337	29197	03433	07035
26	69463	84025	30537	86495	15124	89721	67010	03692
27	27429	18201	87529	61195	48584	45489	29093	07053
28	35997	54613	32898	43843	22322	66033	14547	51447
29	17529	11622	88024	70218	40819	91458	77254	10283
30	91835	07791	13130	23312	13865	80140	43356	57646
31	98341	30885	35193	63277	92726	64287	70330	28724
32	18900	19581	88919	41223	01966	19818	09022	35847
33	31440	97047	22418	72260	04857	99672	98895	96692
34	23815	28377	20004	54032	24869	63361	28030	39562
35	10598	63224	02839	03325	27511	89522	48401	62763

	(9)	(10)	(11)	(12)	(13)	(14)	(15)	(16)
1	44445	77751	36783	10670	81797	02749	86473	96290
2	70857	05590	08260	49295	38767	61355	74651	72889
3	90135	17653	13784	85811	36507	54334	56688	41738
4	59272	62061	82122	90798	67572	34372	43484	28370
5	12123	96619	39040	93921	99368	25513	90211	86578
6	47455	14823	35873	02574	76178	26876	75464	82666
7	44529	05600	68477	97388	59935	41517	39127	35559
8	19930	37601	26357	87502	71973	86193	32224	84097
9	82812	71265	94370	98533	96778	84581	85111	60586
10	99405	37336	63160	91935	64213	38624	90953	25094
11	44225	75782	22483	20512	33651	61610	56071	53581
12	99211	98780	57436	87537	84973	89660	87986	67785
13	60925	82356	66318	74056	83289	67781	34642	99046
14	05118	97802	07334	69331	52779	98287	94425	13356
15	74070	33260	33868	07721	94870	89939	77655	10434
16	88719	35091	14323	73692	24751	02309	57829	02029
17	01017	40500	76085	84306	24633	27079	99705	29751
18	41233	07039	15434	94012	05326	26212	07368	95748
19	59472	57588	03470	70695	47527	97477	81129	52598
20	32568	11804	42642	57319	14113	16824	59348	15130
21	73676	51785	15788	98309	78864	15493	28061	20098
22	22532	43495	30462	44211	86059	54183	39959	45532
23	11771	59781	16227	75651	57258	13708	28249	89826
24	25512	87244	63498	55977	04068	39198	71107	77744
25	90984	03247	76053	86200	18741	20466	06298	57625
26	80314	53113	01836	66373	07296	58148	11905	19067
27	17929	44484	11070	91540	74544	39320	81366	00056
28	42916	61216	56033	46984	00415	43492	41080	07751
29	63092	33485	93951	98185	53952	16602	55810	34266
30	69715	73999	00639	77011	32147	28897	12430	66428
31	89733	23501	57968	64278	79173	55687	80686	22089
32	16903	36720	85425	33670	96564	42857	41421	59656
33	76342	51725	74193	46646	68327	30004	97264	54394
34	20355	14256	47757	52502	43153	60187	18930	49238
35	00040	93251	13516	79213	48938	94203	17654	65841

Appendix G

Transformation of *r* to *z*

$$Z = \frac{1}{2} \log_e \left(\frac{1+r}{1-r} \right)$$

r	Z	r	Z	r	Z	r	Z	r	Z
0.002	0.0020	0.102	0.1024	0.202	0.2048	0.302	0.3117	0.402	0.4260
0.004	0.0040	0.104	0.1044	0.204	0.2069	0.304	0.3139	0.404	0.4284
0.006	0.0060	0.106	0.1064	0.206	0.2090	0.306	0.3161	0.406	0.4308
0.008	0.0080	0.108	0.1084	0.208	0.2111	0.308	0.3183	0.408	0.4332
0.010	0.0100	0.110	0.1104	0.210	0.2132	0.310	0.3205	0.410	0.4356
0.012	0.0120	0.112	0.1125	0.212	0.2153	0.312	0.3228	0.412	0.4380
0.014	0.0140	0.114	0.1145	0.214	0.2174	0.314	0.3250	0.414	0.4404
0.016	0.0160	0.116	0.1165	0.216	0.2195	0.316	0.3272	0.416	0.4428
0.018	0.0180	0.118	0.1186	0.218	0.2216	0.318	0.3294	0.418	0.4453
0.020	0.0200	0.120	0.1206	0.220	0.2237	0.320	0.3316	0.420	0.4477
0.022	0.0220	0.122	0.1226	0.222	0.2258	0.322	0.3339	0.422	0.4501
0.024	0.0240	0.124	0.1246	0.224	0.2279	0.324	0.3361	0.424	0.4526
0.026	0.0260	0.126	0.1267	0.226	0.2300	0.326	0.3383	0.426	0.4550
0.028	0.0280	0.128	0.1287	0.228	0.2321	0.328	0.3406	0.428	0.4574
0.030	0.0300	0.130	0.1307	0.230	0.2342	0.330	0.3428	0.430	0.4599
0.032	0.0320	0.132	0.1328	0.232	0.2363	0.332	0.3451	0.432	0.4624
0.034	0.0340	0.134	0.1348	0.234	0.2384	0.334	0.3473	0.434	0.4648
0.036	0.0360	0.136	0.1368	0.236	0.2405	0.336	0.3496	0.436	0.4673
0.038	0.0380	0.138	0.1389	0.238	0.2427	0.338	0.3518	0.438	0.4698
0.040	0.0400	0.140	0.1409	0.240	0.2448	0.340	0.3541	0.440	0.4722
0.042	0.0420	0.142	0.1430	0.242	0.2469	0.342	0.3564	0.442	0.4747
0.044	0.0440	0.144	0.1450	0.244	0.2490	0.344	0.3586	0.444	0.4772
0.046	0.0460	0.146	0.1471	0.246	0.2512	0.346	0.3609	0.446	0.4797
0.048	0.0480	0.148	0.1491	0.248	0.2533	0.348	0.3632	0.448	0.4822
0.050	0.0500	0.150	0.1511	0.250	0.2554	0.350	0.3654	0.450	0.4847

r	Z	r	Z	r	Z	r	Z	r	Z
0.052	0.0520	0.152	0.1532	0.252	0.2575	0.352	0.3677	0.452	0.4872
0.054	0.0541	0.154	0.1552	0.254	0.2597	0.354	0.3700	0.454	0.4897
0.056	0.0561	0.156	0.1573	0.256	0.2618	0.356	0.3723	0.456	0.4922
0.058	0.0581	0.158	0.1593	0.258	0.2640	0.358	0.3746	0.458	0.4948
0.060	0.0601	0.160	0.1614	0.260	0.2661	0.360	0.3769	0.460	0.4973
0.062	0.0621	0.162	0.1634	0.262	0.2683	0.362	0.3792	0.462	0.4999
0.064	0.0641	0.164	0.1655	0.264	0.2704	0.364	0.3815	0.464	0.5024
0.066	0.0661	0.166	0.1676	0.266	0.2726	0.366	0.3838	0.466	0.5049
0.068	0.0681	0.168	0.1696	0.268	0.2747	0.368	0.3861	0.468	0.5075
0.070	0.0701	0.170	0.1717	0.270	0.2769	0.370	0.3884	0.470	0.5101
0.072	0.0721	0.172	0.1737	0.272	0.2790	0.372	0.3907	0.472	0.5126
0.074	0.0741	0.174	0.1758	0.274	0.2812	0.374	0.3931	0.474	0.5152
0.076	0.0761	0.176	0.1779	0.276	0.2833	0.376	0.3954	0.476	0.5178
0.078	0.0782	0.178	0.1799	0.278	0.2855	0.378	0.3977	0.478	0.5204
0.080	0.0802	0.180	0.1820	0.280	0.2877	0.380	0.4001	0.480	0.5230
0.082	0.0822	0.182	0.1841	0.282	0.2899	0.382	0.4024	0.482	0.5256
0.084	0.0842	0.184	0.1861	0.284	0.2920	0.384	0.4047	0.484	0.5282
0.086	0.0862	0.186	0.1882	0.286	0.2942	0.386	0.4071	0.486	0.5308
0.088	0.0882	0.188	0.1903	0.288	0.2964	0.388	0.4094	0.488	0.5334
0.090	0.0902	0.190	0.1923	0.290	0.2986	0.390	0.4118	0.490	0.5361
0.092	0.0923	0.192	0.1944	0.292	0.3008	0.392	0.4142	0.492	0.5387
0.094	0.0943	0.194	0.1965	0.294	0.3029	0.394	0.4165	0.494	0.5413
0.096	0.0963	0.196	0.1986	0.296	0.3051	0.396	0.4189	0.496	0.5440
0.098	0.0983	0.198	0.2007	0.298	0.3073	0.398	0.4213	0.498	0.5466
0.100	0.1003	0.200	0.2027	0.300	0.3095	0.400	0.4236	0.500	0.5493

Appendix H

Poisson values

x	0.1	0.2	0.3	0.4	0.5	0.6	0.7	0.8	0.9	1.0
0	0.905	0.819	0.741	0.670	0.607	0.549	0.497	0.449	0.407	0.368
1	0.995	0.982	0.963	0.938	0.910	0.878	0.844	0.809	0.772	0.736
2	1.000	0.999	0.996	0.992	0.986	0.977	0.966	0.953	0.937	0.920
3	1.000	1.000	1.000	0.999	0.998	0.997	0.994	0.991	0.987	0.981
4	1.000	1.000	1.000	1.000	1.000	1.000	0.999	0.999	0.998	0.996
5	1.000	1.000	1.000	1.000	1.000	1.000	1.000	1.000	1.000	0.999
6	1.000	1.000	1.000	1.000	1.000	1.000	1.000	1.000	1.000	1.000

x	1.1	1.2	1.3	1.4	1.5	1.6	1.7	1.8	1.9	2.0
0	0.333	0.301	0.273	0.247	0.223	0.202	0.183	0.165	0.150	0.135
1	0.699	0.663	0.627	0.592	0.558	0.525	0.493	0.463	0.434	0.406
2	0.900	0.879	0.857	0.833	0.809	0.783	0.757	0.731	0.704	0.677
3	0.974	0.966	0.957	0.946	0.934	0.921	0.907	0.891	0.875	0.857
4	0.995	0.992	0.989	0.986	0.981	0.976	0.970	0.964	0.956	0.947
5	0.999	0.998	0.998	0.997	0.996	0.994	0.992	0.990	0.987	0.983
6	1.000	1.000	1.000	0.999	0.999	0.999	0.998	0.997	0.997	0.995
7	1.000	1.000	1.000	1.000	1.000	1.000	1.000	0.999	0.999	0.999
8	1.000	1.000	1.000	1.000	1.000	1.000	1.000	1.000	1.000	1.000

x	2.2	2.4	2.6	2.8	3.0	3.2	3.4	3.6	3.8	4.0
0	0.111	0.091	0.074	0.061	0.050	0.041	0.033	0.027	0.022	0.018
1	0.355	0.308	0.267	0.231	0.199	0.171	0.147	0.126	0.107	0.092
2	0.623	0.570	0.518	0.469	0.423	0.380	0.340	0.303	0.269	0.238
3	0.819	0.779	0.736	0.692	0.647	0.603	0.558	0.515	0.473	0.433
4	0.928	0.904	0.877	0.848	0.815	0.781	0.744	0.706	0.668	0.629
5	0.975	0.964	0.951	0.935	0.916	0.895	0.871	0.844	0.816	0.785
6	0.993	0.988	0.983	0.976	0.966	0.955	0.942	0.927	0.909	0.889
7	0.998	0.997	0.995	0.992	0.988	0.983	0.977	0.969	0.960	0.949
8	1.000	0.999	0.999	0.998	0.996	0.994	0.992	0.988	0.984	0.979
9	1.000	1.000	1.000	0.999	0.999	0.998	0.997	0.996	0.994	0.992
10	1.000	1.000	1.000	1.000	1.000	1.000	0.999	0.999	0.998	0.997
11	1.000	1.000	1.000	1.000	1.000	1.000	1.000	1.000	0.999	0.999
12	1.000	1.000	1.000	1.000	1.000	1.000	1.000	1.000	1.000	1.000

x	4.2	4.4	4.6	4.8	5.0	5.2	5.4	5.6	5.8	6.0
0	0.015	0.012	0.010	0.008	0.007	0.006	0.005	0.004	0.003	0.002
1	0.078	0.066	0.056	0.048	0.040	0.034	0.029	0.024	0.021	0.017
2	0.210	0.185	0.163	0.143	0.125	0.109	0.095	0.082	0.072	0.062
3	0.395	0.359	0.326	0.294	0.265	0.238	0.213	0.191	0.170	0.151
4	0.590	0.551	0.513	0.476	0.440	0.406	0.373	0.342	0.313	0.285
5	0.753	0.720	0.686	0.651	0.616	0.581	0.546	0.512	0.478	0.446
6	0.867	0.844	0.818	0.791	0.762	0.732	0.702	0.670	0.638	0.606
7	0.936	0.921	0.905	0.887	0.867	0.845	0.822	0.797	0.771	0.744
8	0.972	0.964	0.955	0.944	0.932	0.918	0.903	0.886	0.867	0.847
9	0.989	0.985	0.980	0.975	0.968	0.960	0.951	0.941	0.929	0.916
10	0.996	0.994	0.992	0.990	0.986	0.982	0.977	0.972	0.965	0.957
11	0.999	0.998	0.997	0.996	0.995	0.993	0.990	0.988	0.984	0.980
12	1.000	0.999	0.999	0.999	0.998	0.997	0.996	0.995	0.993	0.991
13	1.000	1.000	1.000	1.000	0.999	0.999	0.999	0.998	0.997	0.996
14	1.000	1.000	1.000	1.000	1.000	1.000	1.000	0.999	0.999	0.999
15	1.000	1.000	1.000	1.000	1.000	1.000	1.000	1.000	1.000	0.999
16	1.000	1.000	1.000	1.000	1.000	1.000	1.000	1.000	1.000	1.000

x	6.5	7.0	7.5	8.0	8.5	9.0	9.5	10.0	10.5	11.0
0	0.002	0.001	0.001	0.000	0.000	0.000	0.000	0.000	0.000	0.000
1	0.011	0.007	0.005	0.003	0.002	0.001	0.001	0.000	0.000	0.000
2	0.043	0.030	0.020	0.014	0.009	0.006	0.004	0.003	0.002	0.001
3	0.112	0.082	0.059	0.042	0.030	0.021	0.015	0.010	0.007	0.005
4	0.224	0.173	0.132	0.100	0.074	0.055	0.040	0.029	0.021	0.015
5	0.369	0.301	0.241	0.191	0.150	0.116	0.089	0.067	0.050	0.038
6	0.527	0.450	0.378	0.313	0.256	0.207	0.165	0.130	0.102	0.079
7	0.673	0.599	0.525	0.453	0.386	0.324	0.269	0.220	0.179	0.143
8	0.792	0.729	0.662	0.593	0.523	0.456	0.392	0.333	0.279	0.232
9	0.877	0.830	0.776	0.717	0.653	0.587	0.522	0.458	0.397	0.341
10	0.933	0.901	0.862	0.816	0.763	0.706	0.645	0.583	0.521	0.460
11	0.966	0.947	0.921	0.888	0.849	0.803	0.752	0.697	0.639	0.579
12	0.984	0.973	0.957	0.936	0.909	0.876	0.836	0.792	0.742	0.689
13	0.993	0.987	0.978	0.966	0.949	0.926	0.898	0.864	0.825	0.781
14	0.997	0.994	0.990	0.983	0.973	0.959	0.940	0.917	0.888	0.854
15	0.999	0.998	0.995	0.992	0.986	0.978	0.967	0.951	0.932	0.907
16	1.000	0.999	0.998	0.996	0.993	0.989	0.982	0.973	0.960	0.944
17	1.000	1.000	0.999	0.998	0.997	0.995	0.991	0.986	0.978	0.968
18	1.000	1.000	1.000	0.999	0.999	0.998	0.996	0.993	0.988	0.982
19	1.000	1.000	1.000	1.000	0.999	0.999	0.998	0.997	0.994	0.991
20	1.000	1.000	1.000	1.000	1.000	1.000	0.999	0.998	0.997	0.995
21	1.000	1.000	1.000	1.000	1.000	1.000	1.000	0.999	0.999	0.998
22	1.000	1.000	1.000	1.000	1.000	1.000	1.000	1.000	0.999	0.999
23	1.000	1.000	1.000	1.000	1.000	1.000	1.000	1.000	1.000	1.000

Appendix I

χ^2 Values

DF	0.999	0.995	0.99	97.5	0.95	0.90
1	0.000	0.000	0.000	0.001	0.004	0.016
2	0.002	0.010	0.020	0.051	0.103	0.211
3	0.024	0.072	0.115	0.216	0.352	0.584
4	0.091	0.207	0.297	0.484	0.711	1.064
5	0.210	0.412	0.554	0.831	1.145	1.610
6	0.381	0.676	0.872	1.237	1.635	2.204
7	0.598	0.989	1.239	1.690	2.167	2.833
8	0.857	1.344	1.646	2.180	2.733	3.490
9	1.152	1.735	2.088	2.700	3.325	4.168
10	1.479	2.156	2.558	3.247	3.940	4.865
11	1.834	2.603	3.053	3.816	4.575	5.578
12	2.214	3.074	3.571	4.404	5.226	6.304
13	2.617	3.565	4.107	5.009	5.892	7.042
14	3.041	4.075	4.660	5.629	6.571	7.790
15	3.483	4.601	5.229	6.262	7.261	8.547
16	3.942	5.142	5.812	6.908	7.962	9.312
17	4.416	5.697	6.408	7.564	8.672	10.085
18	4.905	6.265	7.015	8.231	9.390	10.865
19	5.407	6.844	7.633	8.907	10.117	11.651
20	5.921	7.434	8.260	9.591	10.851	12.443
21	6.447	8.034	8.897	10.283	11.591	13.240
22	6.983	8.643	9.542	10.982	12.338	14.041
23	7.529	9.260	10.196	11.689	13.091	14.848
24	8.085	9.886	10.856	12.401	13.848	15.659
25	8.649	10.520	11.524	13.120	14.611	16.473
26	9.222	11.160	12.198	13.844	15.379	17.292
27	9.803	11.808	12.879	14.573	16.151	18.114
28	10.391	12.461	13.565	15.308	16.928	18.939
29	10.986	13.121	14.256	16.047	17.708	19.768
30	11.588	13.787	14.953	16.791	18.493	20.599
35	14.688	17.192	18.509	20.569	22.465	24.797
40	17.916	20.707	22.164	24.433	26.509	29.051
45	21.251	24.311	25.901	28.366	30.612	33.350
50	24.674	27.991	29.707	32.357	34.764	37.689
55	28.173	31.735	33.570	36.398	38.958	42.060
60	31.738	35.534	37.485	40.482	43.188	46.459

DF	0.1	0.05	0.025	0.01	0.005	0.001
1	2.706	3.841	5.024	6.635	7.879	10.828
2	4.605	5.991	7.378	9.210	10.597	13.816
3	6.251	7.815	9.348	11.345	12.838	16.266
4	7.779	9.488	11.143	13.277	14.860	18.467
5	9.236	11.070	12.833	15.086	16.750	20.515
6	10.645	12.592	14.449	16.812	18.548	22.458
7	12.017	14.067	16.013	18.475	20.278	24.322
8	13.362	15.507	17.535	20.090	21.955	26.125
9	14.684	16.919	19.023	21.666	23.589	27.877
10	15.987	18.307	20.483	23.209	25.188	29.588
11	17.275	19.675	21.920	24.725	26.757	31.264
12	18.549	21.026	23.337	26.217	28.300	32.910
13	19.812	22.362	24.736	27.688	29.819	34.528
14	21.064	23.685	26.119	29.141	31.319	36.123
15	22.307	24.996	27.488	30.578	32.801	37.697
16	23.542	26.296	28.845	32.000	34.267	39.252
17	24.769	27.587	30.191	33.409	35.718	40.790
18	25.989	28.869	31.526	34.805	37.156	42.312
19	27.204	30.144	32.852	36.191	38.582	43.820
20	28.412	31.410	34.170	37.566	39.997	45.315
21	29.615	32.671	35.479	38.932	41.401	46.797
22	30.813	33.924	36.781	40.289	42.796	48.268
23	32.007	35.172	38.076	41.638	44.181	49.728
24	33.196	36.415	39.364	42.980	45.559	51.179
25	34.382	37.652	40.646	44.314	46.928	52.620
26	35.563	38.885	41.923	45.642	48.290	54.052
27	36.741	40.113	43.195	46.963	49.645	55.476
28	37.916	41.337	44.461	48.278	50.993	56.892
29	39.087	42.557	45.722	49.588	52.336	58.301
30	40.256	43.773	46.979	50.892	53.672	59.703
35	46.059	49.802	53.203	57.342	60.275	66.619
40	51.805	55.758	59.342	63.691	66.766	73.402
45	57.505	61.656	65.410	69.957	73.166	80.077
50	63.167	67.505	71.420	76.154	79.490	86.661
55	68.796	73.311	77.380	82.292	85.749	93.168
60	74.397	79.082	83.298	88.379	91.952	99.607

F-values

F-distribution
Five per cent level (light type),
One per cent (dark type)

degrees of freedom

df	1	2	3	4	5	6	7	8	9	10	11	12	14	16	20	24	30	40	50	75	100	200	500	∞
1	161	200	216	225	230	234	237	239	241	242	243	244	245	246	248	249	250	251	252	253	253	254	254	254
	4,052	4,999	5,403	5,625	5,764	5,859	5,928	5,981	6,022	6,056	6,082	6,106	6,142	6,169	6,208	6,234	6,258	6,286	6,302	6,323	6,334	6,352	6,361	6,366
2	18.51	19.00	19.16	19.25	19.30	19.33	19.36	19.37	19.38	19.39	19.40	19.41	19.42	19.43	19.44	19.45	19.46	19.47	19.47	19.48	19.49	19.49	19.50	19.50
	98.49	99.00	99.17	99.25	99.30	99.33	99.34	99.36	99.38	99.40	99.41	99.42	99.43	99.44	99.45	99.46	99.47	99.48	99.48	99.49	99.49	99.49	99.50	99.50
3	10.13	9.55	9.28	9.12	9.01	8.94	8.88	8.84	8.81	8.78	8.76	8.74	8.71	8.69	8.66	8.64	8.62	8.60	8.58	8.57	8.56	8.54	8.54	8.53
	34.12	30.82	29.46	28.71	28.24	27.91	27.67	27.49	27.34	27.23	27.13	27.05	26.92	26.83	26.69	26.60	26.50	26.41	26.35	26.27	26.23	26.18	26.14	26.12
4	7.71	6.94	6.59	6.39	6.26	6.16	6.09	6.04	6.00	5.96	5.93	5.91	5.87	5.84	5.80	5.77	5.74	5.71	5.70	5.68	5.66	5.65	5.64	5.63
	21.20	18.00	16.69	15.98	15.52	15.21	14.98	14.80	14.66	14.54	14.45	14.37	14.24	14.15	14.02	13.93	13.83	13.74	13.69	13.61	13.57	13.52	13.48	13.46
5	6.61	5.79	5.41	5.19	5.05	4.95	4.88	4.82	4.78	4.74	4.70	4.68	4.64	4.60	4.56	4.53	4.50	4.46	4.44	4.42	4.40	4.38	4.37	4.36
	16.26	13.27	12.06	11.39	10.97	10.67	10.45	10.27	10.15	10.05	9.96	9.89	9.77	9.68	9.55	9.47	9.38	9.29	9.24	9.17	9.13	9.07	9.04	9.02
6	5.99	5.14	4.76	4.53	4.39	4.28	4.21	4.15	4.10	4.06	4.03	4.00	3.96	3.92	3.87	3.84	3.81	3.77	3.75	3.72	3.71	3.69	3.68	3.67
	13.74	10.92	9.78	9.15	8.75	8.47	8.26	8.10	7.98	7.87	7.79	7.72	7.60	7.52	7.39	7.31	7.23	7.14	7.09	7.02	6.99	6.94	6.90	6.88
7	5.59	4.74	4.35	4.12	3.97	3.87	3.79	3.73	3.68	3.63	3.60	3.57	3.52	3.49	3.44	3.41	3.38	3.34	3.32	3.29	3.28	3.25	3.24	3.23
	12.25	9.55	8.45	7.85	7.46	7.19	7.00	6.84	6.71	6.62	6.54	6.47	6.35	6.27	6.15	6.07	5.98	5.90	5.85	5.78	5.75	5.70	5.67	5.65
8	5.32	4.46	4.07	3.84	3.69	3.58	3.50	3.44	3.39	3.34	3.31	3.28	3.23	3.20	3.15	3.12	3.08	3.05	3.03	3.00	2.98	2.96	2.94	2.93
	11.26	8.65	7.59	7.01	6.63	6.37	6.19	6.03	5.91	5.82	5.74	5.67	5.56	5.48	5.36	5.28	5.20	5.11	5.06	5.00	4.96	4.91	4.88	4.86
9	5.12	4.26	3.86	3.63	3.48	3.37	3.29	3.23	3.18	3.13	3.10	3.07	3.02	2.98	2.93	2.90	2.86	2.82	2.80	2.77	2.76	2.73	2.72	2.71
	10.56	8.02	6.99	6.42	6.06	5.80	5.62	5.47	5.35	5.26	5.18	5.11	5.00	4.92	4.80	4.73	4.64	4.56	4.51	4.45	4.41	4.36	4.33	4.31
10	4.96	4.10	3.71	3.48	3.33	3.22	3.14	3.07	3.02	2.97	2.94	2.91	2.86	2.82	2.77	2.74	2.70	2.67	2.64	2.61	2.59	2.56	2.55	2.54
	10.04	7.56	6.55	5.99	5.64	5.39	5.21	5.06	4.95	4.85	4.78	4.71	4.60	4.52	4.41	4.33	4.25	4.17	4.12	4.05	4.01	3.96	3.93	3.91
11	4.84	3.98	3.59	3.36	3.20	3.09	3.01	2.95	2.90	2.86	2.82	2.79	2.74	2.70	2.65	2.61	2.57	2.53	2.50	2.47	2.45	2.42	2.41	2.40
	9.65	7.20	6.22	5.67	5.32	5.07	4.88	4.74	4.63	4.54	4.46	4.40	4.29	4.21	4.10	4.02	3.94	3.86	3.80	3.74	3.70	3.66	3.62	3.60
12	4.75	3.88	3.49	3.26	3.11	3.00	2.92	2.85	2.80	2.76	2.72	2.69	2.64	2.60	2.54	2.50	2.46	2.42	2.40	2.36	2.35	2.32	2.31	2.30
	9.33	6.93	5.95	5.41	5.06	4.82	4.65	4.50	4.39	4.30	4.22	4.16	4.05	3.98	3.86	3.78	3.70	3.61	3.56	3.49	3.46	3.41	3.38	3.36
13	4.67	3.80	3.41	3.18	3.02	2.92	2.84	2.77	2.72	2.67	2.63	2.60	2.55	2.51	2.46	2.42	2.38	2.34	2.32	2.28	2.26	2.24	2.22	2.21
	9.07	6.70	5.74	5.20	4.86	4.62	4.44	4.30	4.19	4.10	4.02	3.96	3.85	3.78	3.67	3.59	3.51	3.42	3.37	3.30	3.27	3.21	3.18	3.16

degrees of freedom

degrees of freedom

df	α	500	200	100	75	50	40	30	24	20	16	14	12	11	10	9	8	7	6	5	4	3	2	1
14	2.13/3.00	2.14/3.02	2.16/3.06	2.19/3.11	2.21/3.14	2.24/3.21	2.27/3.26	2.31/3.34	2.35/3.43	2.39/3.51	2.44/3.62	2.48/3.70	2.53/3.80	2.56/3.86	2.60/3.94	2.65/4.03	2.70/4.14	2.77/4.28	2.85/4.46	2.96/4.69	3.11/5.03	3.34/5.56	3.74/6.51	4.60/8.86
15	2.07/2.87	2.08/2.89	2.10/2.92	2.12/2.97	2.15/3.00	2.18/3.07	2.21/3.12	2.25/3.20	2.29/3.29	2.33/3.36	2.39/3.48	2.43/3.56	2.48/3.67	2.51/3.73	2.55/3.80	2.59/3.89	2.64/4.00	2.70/4.14	2.79/4.32	2.90/4.56	3.06/4.89	3.29/5.42	3.68/6.36	4.54/8.68
16	2.01/2.75	2.02/2.77	2.04/2.80	2.07/2.86	2.09/2.89	2.13/2.96	2.16/3.01	2.20/3.10	2.24/3.18	2.28/3.25	2.33/3.37	2.37/3.45	2.42/3.55	2.45/3.61	2.49/3.69	2.54/3.78	2.59/3.89	2.66/4.03	2.74/4.20	2.85/4.44	3.01/4.77	3.24/5.29	3.63/6.23	4.49/8.53
17	1.96/2.65	1.97/2.67	1.99/2.70	2.02/2.76	2.04/2.79	2.08/2.86	2.11/2.92	2.15/3.00	2.19/3.08	2.23/3.16	2.29/3.27	2.33/3.35	2.38/3.45	2.41/3.52	2.45/3.59	2.50/3.68	2.55/3.79	2.62/3.93	2.70/4.10	2.81/4.34	2.96/4.67	3.20/5.18	3.59/6.11	4.45/8.40
18	1.92/2.57	1.93/2.59	1.95/2.62	1.98/2.68	2.00/2.71	2.04/2.78	2.07/2.83	2.11/2.91	2.15/3.00	2.19/3.07	2.25/3.19	2.29/3.27	2.34/3.37	2.37/3.44	2.41/3.51	2.46/3.60	2.51/3.71	2.58/3.85	2.66/4.01	2.77/4.25	2.93/4.58	3.16/5.09	3.55/6.01	4.41/8.28
19	1.88/2.49	1.90/2.51	1.91/2.54	1.94/2.60	1.96/2.63	2.00/2.70	2.02/2.76	2.07/2.84	2.11/2.92	2.15/3.00	2.21/3.12	2.26/3.19	2.31/3.30	2.34/3.36	2.38/3.43	2.43/3.52	2.48/3.63	2.55/3.77	2.63/3.94	2.74/4.17	2.90/4.50	3.13/5.01	3.52/5.93	4.38/8.18
20	1.84/2.42	1.85/2.44	1.87/2.47	1.90/2.53	1.92/2.56	1.96/2.63	1.99/2.69	2.04/2.77	2.08/2.86	2.12/2.94	2.18/3.05	2.23/3.13	2.28/3.23	2.31/3.30	2.35/3.37	2.40/3.45	2.45/3.56	2.52/3.71	2.60/3.87	2.71/4.10	2.87/4.43	3.10/4.94	3.49/5.85	4.35/8.10
21	1.81/2.36	1.82/2.38	1.84/2.42	1.87/2.47	1.89/2.51	1.93/2.58	1.96/2.63	2.00/2.72	2.05/2.80	2.09/2.88	2.15/2.99	2.20/3.07	2.25/3.17	2.28/3.24	2.32/3.31	2.37/3.40	2.42/3.51	2.49/3.65	2.57/3.81	2.68/4.04	2.84/4.37	3.07/4.87	3.47/5.78	4.32/8.02
22	1.78/2.31	1.80/2.33	1.81/2.37	1.84/2.42	1.87/2.46	1.91/2.53	1.93/2.58	1.98/2.67	2.03/2.75	2.07/2.83	2.13/2.94	2.18/3.02	2.23/3.12	2.26/3.18	2.30/3.26	2.35/3.35	2.40/3.45	2.47/3.59	2.55/3.76	2.66/3.99	2.82/4.31	3.05/4.82	3.44/5.72	4.30/7.94
23	1.76/2.26	1.77/2.28	1.79/2.32	1.82/2.37	1.84/2.41	1.88/2.48	1.91/2.53	1.96/2.62	2.00/2.70	2.04/2.78	2.10/2.89	2.14/2.97	2.20/3.07	2.24/3.14	2.28/3.21	2.32/3.30	2.38/3.41	2.45/3.54	2.53/3.71	2.64/3.94	2.80/4.26	3.03/4.76	3.42/5.66	4.28/7.88
24	1.73/2.21	1.74/2.23	1.76/2.27	1.80/2.33	1.82/2.36	1.86/2.44	1.89/2.49	1.94/2.58	1.98/2.66	2.02/2.74	2.09/2.85	2.13/2.93	2.18/3.03	2.22/3.09	2.26/3.17	2.30/3.25	2.36/3.36	2.43/3.50	2.51/3.67	2.62/3.90	2.78/4.22	3.01/4.72	3.40/5.61	4.26/7.82
25	1.71/2.17	1.72/2.19	1.74/2.23	1.77/2.29	1.80/2.32	1.84/2.40	1.87/2.45	1.92/2.54	1.96/2.62	2.00/2.70	2.06/2.81	2.11/2.89	2.16/2.99	2.20/3.05	2.24/3.13	2.28/3.21	2.34/3.32	2.41/3.46	2.49/3.63	2.60/3.86	2.76/4.18	2.99/4.68	3.38/5.57	4.24/7.77
26	1.69/2.13	1.70/2.15	1.72/2.19	1.76/2.25	1.78/2.28	1.82/2.36	1.85/2.41	1.90/2.50	1.95/2.58	1.99/2.66	2.05/2.77	2.10/2.86	2.15/2.96	2.18/3.02	2.22/3.09	2.27/3.17	2.32/3.29	2.39/3.42	2.47/3.59	2.59/3.82	2.74/4.14	2.98/4.64	3.37/5.53	4.22/7.72

degrees of freedom

**Five per cent level (light type),
One per cent (dark type)**

degrees of freedom

df	1	2	3	4	5	6	7	8	9	10	11	12	14	16	20	24	30	40	50	75	100	200	500	∞
27	4.21 / 7.68	3.35 / 5.49	2.96 / 4.60	2.73 / 4.11	2.57 / 3.79	2.46 / 3.56	2.37 / 3.39	2.30 / 3.26	2.25 / 3.14	2.20 / 3.06	2.16 / 2.98	2.13 / 2.93	2.08 / 2.83	2.03 / 2.74	1.97 / 2.63	1.93 / 2.55	1.88 / 2.47	1.84 / 2.38	1.80 / 2.33	1.76 / 2.25	1.74 / 2.21	1.71 / 2.16	1.68 / 2.12	1.67 / 2.10
28	4.20 / 7.64	3.34 / 5.45	2.95 / 4.57	2.71 / 4.07	2.56 / 3.76	2.44 / 3.53	2.36 / 3.36	2.29 / 3.23	2.24 / 3.11	2.19 / 3.03	2.15 / 2.95	2.12 / 2.90	2.06 / 2.80	2.02 / 2.71	1.96 / 2.60	1.91 / 2.52	1.87 / 2.44	1.81 / 2.35	1.78 / 2.30	1.75 / 2.22	1.72 / 2.18	1.69 / 2.13	1.67 / 2.09	1.65 / 2.06
29	4.18 / 7.60	3.33 / 5.42	2.93 / 4.54	2.70 / 4.04	2.54 / 3.73	2.43 / 3.50	2.35 / 3.33	2.28 / 3.20	2.22 / 3.08	2.18 / 3.00	2.14 / 2.92	2.10 / 2.87	2.05 / 2.77	2.00 / 2.68	1.94 / 2.57	1.90 / 2.49	1.85 / 2.41	1.80 / 2.32	1.77 / 2.27	1.73 / 2.19	1.71 / 2.15	1.68 / 2.10	1.65 / 2.06	1.64 / 2.03
30	4.17 / 7.56	3.32 / 5.39	2.92 / 4.51	2.69 / 4.02	2.53 / 3.70	2.42 / 3.47	2.34 / 3.30	2.27 / 3.17	2.21 / 3.06	2.16 / 2.98	2.12 / 2.90	2.09 / 2.84	2.04 / 2.74	1.99 / 2.66	1.93 / 2.55	1.89 / 2.47	1.84 / 2.38	1.79 / 2.29	1.76 / 2.24	1.72 / 2.16	1.69 / 2.13	1.66 / 2.07	1.64 / 2.03	1.62 / 2.01
32	4.15 / 7.50	3.30 / 5.34	2.90 / 4.46	2.67 / 3.97	2.51 / 3.66	2.40 / 3.42	2.32 / 3.25	2.25 / 3.12	2.19 / 3.01	2.14 / 2.94	2.10 / 2.86	2.07 / 2.80	2.02 / 2.70	1.97 / 2.62	1.91 / 2.51	1.86 / 2.42	1.82 / 2.34	1.76 / 2.25	1.74 / 2.20	1.69 / 2.12	1.67 / 2.08	1.64 / 2.02	1.61 / 1.98	1.59 / 1.96
34	4.13 / 7.44	3.28 / 5.29	2.88 / 4.42	2.65 / 3.93	2.49 / 3.61	2.38 / 3.38	2.30 / 3.21	2.23 / 3.08	2.17 / 2.97	2.12 / 2.89	2.08 / 2.82	2.05 / 2.76	2.00 / 2.66	1.95 / 2.58	1.89 / 2.47	1.84 / 2.38	1.80 / 2.30	1.74 / 2.21	1.71 / 2.15	1.67 / 2.08	1.64 / 2.04	1.61 / 1.98	1.59 / 1.94	1.57 / 1.91
36	4.11 / 7.39	3.26 / 5.25	2.86 / 4.38	2.63 / 3.89	2.48 / 3.58	2.36 / 3.35	2.28 / 3.18	2.21 / 3.04	2.15 / 2.94	2.10 / 2.86	2.06 / 2.78	2.03 / 2.72	1.98 / 2.62	1.93 / 2.54	1.87 / 2.43	1.82 / 2.35	1.78 / 2.26	1.72 / 2.17	1.69 / 2.12	1.65 / 2.04	1.62 / 2.00	1.59 / 1.94	1.56 / 1.90	1.55 / 1.87
38	4.10 / 7.35	3.25 / 5.21	2.85 / 4.34	2.62 / 3.86	2.46 / 3.54	2.35 / 3.32	2.26 / 3.15	2.19 / 3.02	2.14 / 2.91	2.09 / 2.82	2.05 / 2.75	2.02 / 2.69	1.96 / 2.59	1.92 / 2.51	1.85 / 2.40	1.80 / 2.32	1.76 / 2.22	1.71 / 2.14	1.67 / 2.08	1.63 / 2.00	1.60 / 1.97	1.57 / 1.90	1.54 / 1.86	1.53 / 1.84
40	4.08 / 7.31	3.23 / 5.18	2.84 / 4.31	2.61 / 3.83	2.45 / 3.51	2.34 / 3.29	2.25 / 3.12	2.18 / 2.99	2.12 / 2.88	2.07 / 2.80	2.04 / 2.73	2.00 / 2.66	1.95 / 2.56	1.90 / 2.49	1.84 / 2.37	1.79 / 2.29	1.74 / 2.20	1.69 / 2.11	1.66 / 2.05	1.61 / 1.97	1.59 / 1.94	1.55 / 1.88	1.53 / 1.84	1.51 / 1.81
42	4.07 / 7.27	3.22 / 5.15	2.83 / 4.29	2.59 / 3.80	2.44 / 3.49	2.32 / 3.26	2.24 / 3.10	2.17 / 2.96	2.11 / 2.86	2.06 / 2.77	2.02 / 2.70	1.99 / 2.64	1.94 / 2.54	1.89 / 2.46	1.82 / 2.35	1.78 / 2.26	1.73 / 2.17	1.68 / 2.08	1.64 / 2.02	1.60 / 1.94	1.57 / 1.91	1.54 / 1.85	1.51 / 1.80	1.49 / 1.78
44	4.06 / 7.24	3.21 / 5.12	2.82 / 4.26	2.58 / 3.78	2.43 / 3.46	2.31 / 3.24	2.23 / 3.07	2.16 / 2.94	2.10 / 2.84	2.05 / 2.75	2.01 / 2.68	1.98 / 2.62	1.92 / 2.52	1.88 / 2.44	1.81 / 2.32	1.76 / 2.24	1.72 / 2.15	1.66 / 2.06	1.63 / 2.00	1.58 / 1.92	1.56 / 1.88	1.52 / 1.82	1.50 / 1.78	1.48 / 1.75
46	4.05 / 7.21	3.20 / 5.10	2.81 / 4.24	2.57 / 3.76	2.42 / 3.44	2.30 / 3.22	2.22 / 3.05	2.14 / 2.92	2.09 / 2.82	2.04 / 2.73	2.00 / 2.66	1.97 / 2.60	1.91 / 2.50	1.87 / 2.42	1.80 / 2.30	1.75 / 2.22	1.71 / 2.13	1.65 / 2.04	1.62 / 1.98	1.57 / 1.90	1.54 / 1.86	1.51 / 1.80	1.48 / 1.76	1.46 / 1.72
48	4.04 / 7.19	3.19 / 5.08	2.80 / 4.22	2.56 / 3.74	2.41 / 3.42	2.30 / 3.20	2.21 / 3.04	2.14 / 2.90	2.08 / 2.80	2.03 / 2.71	1.99 / 2.64	1.96 / 2.58	1.90 / 2.48	1.86 / 2.40	1.79 / 2.28	1.74 / 2.20	1.70 / 2.11	1.64 / 2.02	1.61 / 1.96	1.56 / 1.88	1.53 / 1.84	1.50 / 1.78	1.47 / 1.73	1.45 / 1.70

degrees of freedom

degrees of freedom

df	α	500	200	100	75	50	40	30	24	20	16	14	12	11	10	9	8	7	6	5	4	3	2	1
50	1.44 / 1.68	1.46 / 1.71	1.48 / 1.76	1.52 / 1.82	1.55 / 1.86	1.60 / 1.94	1.63 / 2.00	1.69 / 2.10	1.74 / 2.18	1.78 / 2.26	1.85 / 2.39	1.90 / 2.46	1.95 / 2.56	1.98 / 2.62	2.02 / 2.70	2.07 / 2.78	2.13 / 2.88	2.20 / 3.02	2.29 / 3.18	2.40 / 3.41	2.56 / 3.72	2.79 / 4.20	3.18 / 5.06	4.03 / 7.17
55	1.41 / 1.64	1.43 / 1.66	1.46 / 1.71	1.50 / 1.78	1.52 / 1.82	1.58 / 1.90	1.61 / 1.96	1.67 / 2.06	1.72 / 2.15	1.76 / 2.23	1.83 / 2.35	1.88 / 2.43	1.93 / 2.53	1.97 / 2.59	2.00 / 2.66	2.05 / 2.75	2.11 / 2.85	2.18 / 2.98	2.27 / 3.15	2.38 / 3.37	2.54 / 3.68	2.78 / 4.16	3.17 / 5.01	4.02 / 7.12
60	1.39 / 1.60	1.41 / 1.63	1.44 / 1.68	1.48 / 1.74	1.50 / 1.79	1.56 / 1.87	1.59 / 1.93	1.65 / 2.03	1.70 / 2.12	1.75 / 2.20	1.81 / 2.32	1.86 / 2.40	1.92 / 2.50	1.95 / 2.56	1.99 / 2.63	2.04 / 2.72	2.10 / 2.82	2.17 / 2.95	2.25 / 3.12	2.37 / 3.34	2.52 / 3.65	2.76 / 4.13	3.15 / 4.98	4.00 / 7.08
65	1.37 / 1.56	1.39 / 1.60	1.42 / 1.64	1.46 / 1.71	1.49 / 1.76	1.54 / 1.84	1.57 / 1.90	1.63 / 2.00	1.68 / 2.09	1.73 / 2.18	1.80 / 2.30	1.85 / 2.37	1.90 / 2.47	1.94 / 2.54	1.98 / 2.61	2.02 / 2.70	2.08 / 2.79	2.15 / 2.93	2.24 / 3.09	2.36 / 3.31	2.51 / 3.62	2.75 / 4.10	3.14 / 4.95	3.99 / 7.04
70	1.35 / 1.53	1.37 / 1.56	1.40 / 1.62	1.45 / 1.69	1.47 / 1.74	1.53 / 1.82	1.56 / 1.88	1.62 / 1.98	1.67 / 2.07	1.72 / 2.15	1.79 / 2.28	1.84 / 2.35	1.89 / 2.45	1.93 / 2.51	1.97 / 2.59	2.01 / 2.67	2.07 / 2.77	2.14 / 2.91	2.23 / 3.07	2.35 / 3.29	2.50 / 3.60	2.74 / 4.08	3.13 / 4.92	3.98 / 7.01
80	1.32 / 1.49	1.35 / 1.52	1.38 / 1.57	1.42 / 1.65	1.45 / 1.70	1.51 / 1.78	1.54 / 1.84	1.60 / 1.94	1.65 / 2.03	1.70 / 2.11	1.77 / 2.24	1.82 / 2.32	1.88 / 2.41	1.91 / 2.48	1.95 / 2.55	1.99 / 2.64	2.05 / 2.74	2.12 / 2.87	2.21 / 3.04	2.33 / 3.25	2.48 / 3.56	2.72 / 4.04	3.11 / 4.88	3.96 / 6.96
100	1.28 / 1.43	1.30 / 1.46	1.34 / 1.51	1.39 / 1.59	1.42 / 1.64	1.48 / 1.73	1.51 / 1.79	1.57 / 1.89	1.63 / 1.98	1.68 / 2.06	1.75 / 2.19	1.79 / 2.26	1.85 / 2.36	1.88 / 2.43	1.92 / 2.51	1.97 / 2.59	2.03 / 2.69	2.10 / 2.82	2.19 / 2.99	2.30 / 3.20	2.46 / 3.51	2.70 / 3.98	3.09 / 4.82	3.94 / 6.90
125	1.25 / 1.37	1.27 / 1.40	1.31 / 1.46	1.36 / 1.54	1.39 / 1.59	1.45 / 1.68	1.49 / 1.75	1.55 / 1.85	1.60 / 1.94	1.65 / 2.03	1.72 / 2.15	1.77 / 2.23	1.83 / 2.33	1.86 / 2.40	1.90 / 2.47	1.95 / 2.56	2.01 / 2.65	2.08 / 2.79	2.17 / 2.95	2.29 / 3.17	2.44 / 3.47	2.68 / 3.94	3.07 / 4.78	3.92 / 6.84
150	1.22 / 1.33	1.25 / 1.37	1.29 / 1.43	1.34 / 1.51	1.37 / 1.56	1.44 / 1.66	1.47 / 1.72	1.54 / 1.83	1.59 / 1.91	1.64 / 2.00	1.71 / 2.12	1.76 / 2.20	1.82 / 2.30	1.85 / 2.37	1.89 / 2.44	1.94 / 2.53	2.00 / 2.62	2.07 / 2.76	2.16 / 2.92	2.27 / 3.14	2.43 / 3.44	2.67 / 3.91	3.06 / 4.75	3.91 / 6.81
200	1.19 / 1.28	1.22 / 1.33	1.26 / 1.39	1.32 / 1.48	1.35 / 1.53	1.42 / 1.62	1.45 / 1.69	1.52 / 1.79	1.57 / 1.88	1.62 / 1.97	1.69 / 2.09	1.74 / 2.17	1.80 / 2.28	1.83 / 2.34	1.87 / 2.41	1.92 / 2.50	1.98 / 2.60	2.05 / 2.73	2.14 / 2.90	2.26 / 3.11	2.41 / 3.41	2.65 / 3.88	3.04 / 4.71	3.89 / 6.76
400	1.13 / 1.19	1.16 / 1.24	1.22 / 1.32	1.28 / 1.42	1.32 / 1.47	1.38 / 1.57	1.42 / 1.64	1.49 / 1.74	1.54 / 1.84	1.60 / 1.92	1.67 / 2.04	1.72 / 2.12	1.78 / 2.23	1.81 / 2.29	1.85 / 2.37	1.90 / 2.46	1.96 / 2.55	2.03 / 2.69	2.12 / 2.85	2.23 / 3.06	2.39 / 3.36	2.62 / 3.83	3.02 / 4.66	3.86 / 6.70
1000	1.08 / 1.11	1.13 / 1.19	1.19 / 1.28	1.26 / 1.38	1.30 / 1.44	1.36 / 1.54	1.41 / 1.61	1.47 / 1.71	1.53 / 1.81	1.58 / 1.89	1.65 / 2.01	1.70 / 2.09	1.76 / 2.20	1.80 / 2.26	1.84 / 2.34	1.89 / 2.43	1.95 / 2.53	2.02 / 2.66	2.10 / 2.82	2.22 / 3.04	2.38 / 3.34	2.61 / 3.80	3.00 / 4.62	3.85 / 6.66
α	1.00 / 1.00	1.11 / 1.15	1.17 / 1.25	1.24 / 1.36	1.28 / 1.41	1.35 / 1.52	1.40 / 1.59	1.46 / 1.69	1.52 / 1.79	1.57 / 1.87	1.64 / 1.99	1.69 / 2.07	1.75 / 2.18	1.79 / 2.24	1.83 / 2.32	1.88 / 2.41	1.94 / 2.51	2.01 / 2.64	2.09 / 2.80	2.21 / 3.02	2.37 / 3.32	2.60 / 3.78	2.99 / 4.60	3.84 / 6.64

degrees of freedom

Index

abscissa 1, 140
absence from work 135
absolute values 8
AIDS 118
algebraic expressions
  correlation *see* correlation
  prediction equations 166–8
  straight line equations 139–40
    calculating gradients 144–7
    coordinates 140, 141
    going from graph to algebra 147–8
    graphing 140–4
alternative hypothesis 89
ANOVA (analysis of variance) 171–2
  between groups variance 172, 176, 177
  Between Samples Sum of Squares
    (BSS) 181
  double sigma notation 179–81
  normality of parent populations 173,
    174
  practical uses 184
  random assignment 173, 174
  setting up the variance table 178–9
  Total Sum of Squares (TSS) 181
  variance homogeneity of parent
    populations 173, 174–5
  with one-way classification 175
  within groups variance 172, 176, 177–8
  Within Samples Sum of Squares
    (WSS) 181
  worked example 182–3
arithmetic mean 5, 7, 9
arthritis 83

bar graphs 4
bias 83, 84
bimodal distribution 2
binomial distribution 53
  algebraic expression 57–60
  relationship with normal distribution
    62–4

testing statistical hypotheses 60–2
throwing dice 53–7
binomials 26–9
bivariate data 152, 153, 163–6
  see also correlation

cancer tests 118
Cartesian Coordinates 140, 141
cells 131
central tendency 5–7, 9
Chi-Square (χ^2) Test 129–36
  χ^2 values 209–10
class intervals 13, 16
class limits 13
cleft palate 57
clusters 14
coefficients 27
combinations 35–6
conditional probability 114
confidence limits 96–7, 105–6
continuous data 2
correlation 139, 151–2
  computing a value 152–6
  linear correlation 152, 163–6
  Pearson product-moment correlation
    coefficient (r) 151, 156–8, 160–1
    calculating r from grouped data
      158–60
    sampling distribution of r-scores
      161–2
curvilinear correlation 152

data
  distributions 1–5
  grouped 11–16
  measures 5–6
    central tendency 5–7, 9
    dispersion 6, 8–9
  population samples and scores 1
  ungrouped 10–11
dependent events 115–16

Descartes, René 140
descriptive statistics 21
deviation 8
dice throws 53–7
discontinuous (discrete) data 2, 4
dispersion 8–9
distribution-free statistics 121
distributions 1–5
    see also binomial distribution;
        normal distribution; Poisson
        distribution

epidemiology
    conditional probability 114
    definition 109
    dependent and independent events
        115–16
    joint probability 112–14
    mutually exclusive events 116–17
    proportions and rates 109–11
    testing
        predictive value 111, 112
        sensitivity 111, 112
        specificity 111, 112
Everley's syndrome 105, 106
exam scores 130–1
expected values 129, 135

factorial notation 31–2, 34
fiducial limits 96–7, 105–6
Fisher Z-transformations 161–2, 202–5
frequency 1

Gauss, Karl Friedrich 47
genetic illness 25–6, 57
genetics 129
Gossett, William S 99
graphs 140–4
    bivariate data 152, 153
    coordinates 140, 141
    going from graph to algebra 147–8
    straight line equations 139–40
        calculating gradients 144–7
grouped data 11–16

haemophilia 116–17
hare lip 57

health calculations 24–6
height distributions 91–2
histograms 4, 59

incidence 110–11
independent events 71–3, 115–16
inferential statistics 21–2
inherited conditions 25–6, 57
intervals 97
investment advice 118–19
IQ scores 45, 158–9, 166–8

joint probability 112–14

kurtosis 3

leptokurtotic distribution 3
linear correlation 152, 163–6

malaria 59–62, 116
mean 5, 7, 9
median 7, 16
Mendelian genetics 131
menopause 84
midpoints 13, 15
migraine 84
mode 7, 16
mutually exclusive events 116–17

negatively skewed distribution 2
non-parametric statistics 121
    Chi-Square (χ^2) Test 129–36
        χ^2 values 209–10
    Sign Test 125–7
    Wilcoxon two-sample test
        independent samples 121–5, 195–6
        paired cases 127–9, 197–9
normal distribution 3, 43–5
    infinite series 46–7
    relating s to probabilities 47–51
    relationship with binomial
        distribution 62–4
    see also non-parametric statistics
null hypothesis 89–91

observed values 130, 135
one-tailed test 89

ordinate 1, 141

paired cases
    Sign Test 125–7
    small samples 100, 103–7
    Wilcoxon two-sample test 127–9,
        197–9
parameters 9, 43
parametric statistics 43
Pearson product-moment correlation
        coefficient (r) 151, 156–8, 160–1
    calculating r from grouped data
        158–60
    sampling distribution of r-scores
        161–2
percentages 109
permutations 29–31, 32–4
    combinations 35–6
pie-charts 5
placebos 87
platykurtotic distribution 4
Poisson distribution 64–74
    estimation of λ and applications
        74–81
Poisson values 206–8
political attitudes 134
population samples 1
    see also sampling
positively skewed distribution 3
prediction
    linear correlation 152, 163–6
    regression line 166–8
predictive value 111, 112
prevalence 109, 110, 111
probability 22–4
        apparent anomalies 117–19
        binomial distribution 53
        algebraic expression 57–60
        dice throws 53–7
        relationship with normal
            distribution 62–4
        testing statistical hypotheses 60–2
    conditional probability 114
    dependent and independent events
        115–16
    health calculations 24–6
    joint probability 112–14

mutually exclusive events 116–17
    normal distribution 47–51
    Poisson distribution 64–74
    repeated trials 36–9
probability space 26

random events 71–3
random numbers 200–1
random sampling 84–6
    testing a sample 86–8
range 5, 8
regression line 166–8
repeated trials 36–9
research projects
    formulating the research problem
        185–7
    revision 188–9
    writing up the proposal 187–8

sampling
    bias 83, 84
    null hypothesis 89–91
    paired cases
        Sign Test 125–7
        small samples 100, 103–7
        Wilcoxon two-sample test 127–9,
            197–9
    random sampling 84–6
        testing a sample 86–8
    sample means 87–94
        confidence limits 96–7, 105–6
        difference of means of large
            samples 94–6
    small samples
        comparing a sample mean with the
            population mean 106
        establishing an interval for the
            population mean 105–6
        problems 99–100
        t-test 87, 99, 100–5
        two samples 100, 103–7
    two independent samples
        t-test 103–5
        Wilcoxon two-sample test 121–5,
            195–6
scatter diagrams 153, 154, 163, 164
scores 1

sensitivity 111, 112, 135
sickle cell anaemia 90, 116
Sign Test 125–7
significance level 61, 89, 106
social classes 133–4
specificity 111, 112
spread 6
squared deviation 8
standard deviation 8–9, 15, 16–17
   pairs of samples 106–7
   relating s to probabilities 47–51
standard error 88, 94, 95
statistics
   descriptive 21
   inferential 21–2
   non-parametric 121
straight line equations 139–40
   calculating gradients 144–7
   going from graph to algebra
      147–8
   graphing 140–4
Student's t-test 99
sub-acute malaria 59–62

t-test 87, 99, 100–5
   distribution of t 194
temperature readings 100–1

thalassemia 90
tone perception tests 131–2
two-tailed test 89
Type 1/Type 2 error 85, 88

ungrouped data 10–11

variability 93, 107
variables
   correlation *see* correlation
variance 9, 15
Venn Diagrams 112–14

Wilcoxon two-sample test
   independent samples 121–5, 195–6
   paired cases 127–9, 197–9

x-axis 1, 140

y-axis 1, 140

Z-tables 48, 60, 61, 86, 90, 94, 97
   areas under the normal probability
      curve 192–3
   Fisher Z-transformations 161–2,
      202–5
zero factorial 32